BLACK
AMERICAN
HEALTH

Recent Titles in
Bibliographies and Indexes in Afro-American and African Studies

Blacks in the American Armed Forces, 1776-1983: A Bibliography
Lenwood G. Davis and George Hill, compilers

Education of the Black Adult in the United States: An Annotated Bibliography
Leo McGee and Harvey G. Neufeldt, compilers

A Guide to the Archives of Hampton Institute
Fritz J. Malval, compiler

A Bibliographical Guide to Black Studies Programs in the United States: An Annotated Bibliography
Lenwood G. Davis and George Hill, compilers

Wole Soyinka: A Bibliography of Primary and Secondary Sources
James Gibbs, Ketu H. Katrak, and Henry Louis Gates, Jr., compilers

Afro-American Demography and Urban Issues: A Bibliography
R. A. Obudho and Jeannine B. Scott, compilers

Afro-American Reference: An Annotated Bibliography of Selected Resources
Nathaniel Davis, compiler and editor

The Afro-American Short Story: A Comprehensive, Annotated Index with Selected Commentaries
Preston M. Yancy, compiler

Black Labor in America, 1865-1983: A Selected Annotated Bibliography
Joseph Wilson, compiler and editor

Martin Luther King, Jr.: An Annotated Bibliography
Sherman E. Pyatt, compiler

Blacks in the Humanities, 1750-1984: A Selected Annotated Bibliography
Donald Franklin Joyce, compiler

The Black Family in the United States: A Revised, Updated, Selectively Annotated Bibliography
Lenwood G. Davis, compiler

Black American Families, 1965-1984: A Classified, Selectively Annotated Bibliography
Walter R. Allen, editor

Index to Poetry by Black American Women
Dorothy Hilton Chapman, compiler

BLACK AMERICAN HEALTH

An Annotated Bibliography

Compiled by
MITCHELL F. RICE
and
WOODROW JONES, JR.

BIBLIOGRAPHIES AND INDEXES
IN AFRO-AMERICAN AND AFRICAN STUDIES, NUMBER 17

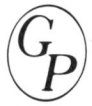

GREENWOOD PRESS
NEW YORK • WESTPORT, CONNECTICUT • LONDON

Library of Congress Cataloging-in-Publicaton Data

Rice, Mitchell F.
 Black American health.

 (Bibliographies and indexes in Afro-American and
African studies, ISSN 0742-6925 ; no. 17)
 Includes bibliographies and index.
 1. Afro-Americans—Health and hygiene—Abstracts.
2. Afro-Americans—Medical care—Abstracts. 3. Social
medicine—United States—Abstracts. I. Jones, Woodrow.
II. Title. III. Series. [DNLM: 1. Blacks—
United States—abstracts. 2. Health—United States—
abstracts. 3. Morbidity—United States—abstracts.
ZWA 900 AA1 R4b]
 RA448.5.N4R53 1987   362.1'08996073   86-25745
 ISBN 0-313-24887-7 (lib. bdg. : alk. paper)

Copyright © 1987 by Mitchell F. Rice and Woodrow Jones, Jr.

All rights reserved. No portion of this book may be
reproduced, by any process or technique, without the
express written consent of the publisher.

Library of Congress Catalog Card Number: 86-25745
ISBN: 0-313-24887-7
ISSN: 0742-6925

First published in 1987

Greenwood Press, Inc.
88 Post Road West, Westport, Connecticut 06881

Printed in the United States of America

The paper used in this book complies with the
Permanent Paper Standard issued by the National
Information Standards Organization (Z39.48-1984).

10 9 8 7 6 5 4 3 2 1

TO THE
GOOD HEALTH OF
BLACK AMERICANS

Contents

Introduction:	Being Black and Unhealthy	ix
1.	Cardiovascular System	3
2.	Mental Health	19
3.	Health Care Problems	52
4.	Assessment Studies	72
5.	Cancer	103
6.	Political/Social Issues	111
7.	Sickle Cell Anemia	124
	Appendix: Black Health Organizations	132
	Author Index	134

Introduction:
Being Black and Unhealthy

Twenty years ago, in 1966, the President of the American Public Health Association remarked that: "Clearly, in terms of health, there is a special disadvantage to being a Negro in the United States which transcends being poor."[1] In 1971 the U.S. Department of Health, Education and Welfare noted that:

> On nearly every index we have, the poor and racial minorities fare worse than their opposites. Their lives are shorter; they have more chronic debilitating illnesses; their infant and maternal death rates are higher; their protection, through immunization against infectious diseases, is far lower. They also have far less access to health services and this is particularly true of poor and nonwhite children, millions of whom receive little or no dental care and pediatric care.[2]

Fourteen years later, in 1985, the U.S. Department of Health and Human Services (DHHS) declared that:

> Despite the unprecedented explosion in scientific knowledge and the phenomenal capacity of medicine to diagnose, treat and cure disease, Blacks...have not fully benefitted equally from the fruits of science or from those systems responsible for translating and using health science technology.[3]

DHHS has further observed that:

> Blacks today have a life expectancy already reached by whites in the early 1950s, or a lag of about 30 years.... In 1960 Blacks suffered 44.3 infant deaths for every 1,000 births, roughly twice the rate for Whites, 22.9. Moreover, in 1981 Blacks suffered 20 infant deaths per 1,000 births, twice the white level of 10.5, but similar to the White rate of 1960.[4]

These observations would seem to support the view that blacks have been, and continue to be, recipients of "second-class medicine."[5] Further, several analysts of black health care note a direct relationship between racism and the prevalence of second-class medicine in the black community.[6] Almost every set of government indexes shows significant health disparities between blacks and whites. The most critical disparities exist in the areas that are commonly accepted as health status indicators: life expectancy, infant mortality, and maternal mortality. General mortality data also shows significant disparities between blacks and whites. In the area of substance abuse, a disproportionate percentage of blacks are chronic users and abusers.

HEALTH STATUS INDICATORS

Life Expectancy

Life expectancy is regarded as a particularly useful indicator for the general health condition of a population group. When life expectancy data first became available at the turn of the century, it showed that blacks were expected to live 33 years as compared to 47.6 years for whites. Although black life expectancy has shown marked improvement from 1900 to recent years, whites still outlive blacks by several years. In 1982 whites outlived blacks by nearly six years, 75.1 to 69.3 years. White men in 1982 outlived black men by nearly seven years, while white men outlived black women by nearly five years.[7]

Infant Mortality

The black infant mortality rate has been consistently double that of the white rate for the last thirty years. While both the black and white infant mortality rates have declined significantly since 1950, the ratio between the two groups in 1980 was virtually the same as it was in 1950.[8] A major contributor to the black infant mortality rate is the problem of low-birthweight infants, who weigh 2,500 grams (5.5 pounds) or less. Blacks are twice as likely as whites to have low-birthweight infants, and two and one half times as likely to have very low-birthweight infants (under 1,500 grams).[9]

Maternal Mortality

Since 1940, the black maternal mortality rate has been about two to three times higher than the rate for whites. In 1940 the black maternal mortality rate was 781.7 per 100,000 live births, compared to 319.8 for whites; in 1950, 223.0 to 61.1; in 1960, 103.6 to 26.0; in 1970, 59.8 to 14.4; and in 1981, 20.4 to 6.3. Several risk factors are associated with maternal mortality and morbidity, including heart disease and diabetes. The prevalence of diabetes is considerably higher among black women than it is among whites.[10]

A significant causal factor is the set of circumstances under which a child is born. In 1940, close to one-half of all black births were attended by a midwife and were outside the hospital setting, compared with only four percent of white births for the same year. By 1950 more than one-fourth of all black babies were

INTRODUCTION   xi

delivered by midwives. By 1972, the rate had finally dropped to one in fifty.[11] In 1980 about 99 percent of black births occurred in hospitals, and nearly 97 percent were attended by physicians.[12] However, adequate prenatal care is still a problem among pregnant black women. In 1980 nearly 10 out of every 100 black expectant mothers, or 9.6 percent, waited until the 7th-9th month to begin prenatal care. About 3.2 percent received no prenatal care at all.[13]

MORTALITY AND BLACKS

In 1980 the death rate for black Americans was 50 percent higher than that for whites for all categories combined. Diseases of the heart are the leading cause of death in the United States. Deaths from coronary heart disease are 50 pecent higher for black males than for white males, and nearly 30 percent higher for black females than for white females. Blacks in comparison to whites have higher mortality rates from other leading causes of death as well. Black mortality rates are significantly higher than whites in the following areas: cancer (malignant neoplasms), cerebrovascular disease, accidents and adverse effects, diabetes, mellitus, and chronic liver disease and cirrhosis.[14] While lifestyles differences to some degree may contribute to the black/white differential in mortality, there are also other factors. Blacks are exposed to more occupational hazards, have far less access to high quality medical care, receive considerably fewer preventative services, and do not seek treatment until the later stages of a disease or illness.[15] Overall, blacks have a higher risk of contracting illnesses and a greater exposure to life-threatening situations. Increased risk is "definitely related to the wide impact of racism" and discrimination.[16]

SUBSTANCE ABUSE

In the area of substance abuse, a disproportionate number of blacks suffer from opiate and alcohol dependency. This fact, coupled with the alarmingly high rate of poverty and unemployment in the black community, makes the negative impact of substance abuse more severe. This high level of abuse has contributed to the overall poor health status of blacks, as medical and social epidemiological data have linked such excesses to an increased risk of premature mortality and morbidity. In this way, substance abuse may be correlated with many of the leading causes of death among blacks.[17]

In conclusion, health status indicators point to a crisis in health care in the black community. Actions and strategies must be designed and implemented whereby blacks can benefit substantially from the health care system in the United States.

PURPOSE OF THIS BOOK

This book presents a comprehensive annotated listing of more than 350 sources relating to black health care. It is divided into seven chapters; Cardiovascular System, Mental Health, Health Care Problems, Assessment Studies, Cancer, Political/Social Issues, and Sickle-Cell Anemia. An appendix listing the names and addresses of black health and health related organizations is located at the end of the book. As political scientists, we find the chapter on "Political/Social Issues" quite appealing. When we attend health conferences we are asked on numerous occasions, "What's a political scientist doing studying health care?" We find that health professionals and practitioners need to be reminded that politics and the political process play a major role in the distribution of valued benefits in society. Good health is indeed a valued societal benefit.

During our research on the accompanying volume, Health Care Issues in Black America (Greenwood Press), we could not locate a comprehensive annotated bibliography in book form on the subject of black health care. This represents our motivation for taking on this work. We have made a conscious effort to include primary sources that were published in the 1970s and 1980s, a time during which a wealth of literature appeared examining black health status, health needs and health problems. We hope this work is viewed as a major reference source for researchers, students and others interested in black health care.

Such a work as this could not have been completed without invaluable assistance. We wish to thank our graduate student assistants, who spent countless hours in the library, and our secretarial staff, whose skills made this work possible. Also, Professor Rice is indebted for research assistance provided by a Rockefeller Postdoctoral Research Fellowship.

NOTES

1. Alonzo Yerby, "The Disadvantaged and Health Care," American Journal of Public Health 56 (1966): 5-9.

2. U.S. Department of Health, Education, and Welfare, Toward A Comprehensive Health Policy for the 1970s: A White Paper (Washington, D.C.: Government Printing Office, 1971).

3. U.S. Department of Health and Human Services, Report of the Secretary's Task Force on Black and Minority Health, Volume I: Executive Summary, (Washington, D.C.: Government Printing Office, 1985), p. 1.

4. Ibid., p. 2.

5. Dorothy K. Newman et.al. Protest Politics and Prosperity: Black Americans and White Institutions, 1940-1975 (New York: Pantheon Books, 1978).

6. See, for example, J.N. Gayles, "Health Brutality and the Black Life Cycle," Black Scholar (May 1972): 2-9 and Richard Cooper et.al. "Racism, Society, and Disease: An Exploration of the Social and Biological Mechanisms of Differential Mortality," International Journal of Health Services 11 (3)(Fall 1981): 389-414.

7. U.S. Department of Health and Human Service, Public Health Service, Health and Prevention Profile, United States 1983 (Washington, D.C.: Government Printing Office, 1983), Table 10, p. 99.

8. U.S. Department of Health and Human Services, Public Health Service, Health Status of Minorities and Low Income Groups (Washington, D.C.: Government Printing Office, 1985): p. 67, Table 5.

9. Dorothy Howze, "The Black Infant Mortality Rate: An Unequal Chance for Life," Urban League Review 9 (Winter 1985/86): 20-25.

10. Health Status of Minorities and Low Income Groups, pp. 51-52.

11. See Mitchell F. Rice, "Black Health Care: Another Look at an Old Problem," Texas Public Health Association Journal 33 (3) (Fall 1981): 17-20 and Anne S. Lee, Maternal Mortality in the United States," Phylon: The Journal of Race and Culture 38 (September 1977): 264-65.

12. Health Status of Minorities and Low Income Groups, Table 19, p. 75.

13. Ibid., Table 18, p. 75.

14. Antonio A. Rene' and Patrick R. Clifford, "Black and White Differentials in Mortality," Urban League Review 9 (Winter 1985/86): 13-19.

15. Mitchell F. Rice and Woodrow Jones, Jr. "Black Health Inequities and the American Health Care System," Health Policy and Education 3 (October 1982): 195-214.

16. "Getting Along," Houston Post (October 26, 1980), p. 30.

17. Patrick R. Clifford and Antonio A. Rene', "Substance Abuse Among Blacks: An Epidemiological Perspective," Urban League Review 9 (Winter 1985/86): 52-57.

BLACK AMERICAN HEALTH

1. Cardiovascular System

1. Ahmed, S. S., Rozefort R. and Brancato, R. "Incidence of Acute Myocardial Infarction Among Blacks in an Urban Community." Journal of the Medical Society of New Jersey 74 (12) (1977): 1058-60.

   A study of the incidence of acute myocardial infarction (AMI) in urban blacks among the residents of Paterson, N.J. treated in hospitals in and around the city. Of the 162 documented cases among Patersonians, 17 were black. The crude rate per 100,000 of AMI among persons over 30 years was higher in whites as a group than in blacks. The age specific rate revealed higher incidence in blacks in the 30 to 39, 70 to 79 and 80 to 89 age groups. Smoking was the most frequent risk factor in the two groups. Blacks, however, had a higher prevalence of hypertension, 63% as compared to 23% in whites. These data indicate that the rate of AMI in age related blacks is actually higher than in whites. Concludes that the reported rarity of AMI in blacks may be due to the fact that the black population is relatively younger.

2. Berenson, G.S. et.al. "Black-White Contrasts as Determinants of Cardiovascular Risk in Childhood: Precursors of Coronary Artery and Primary Hypertensive Diseases." American Heart Journal 108 (9) (1984): 672-83.

   Studies of children have identified black-white differences in anthropometric, hormonal, enzymatic, and renal mechanisms related to the development of coronary artery disease and hypertension. Black children have greater body density, higher blood pressure, higher cholesterol and insulin levels. Whereas white children have a higher percentage of body fat a faster heart rate, high hemoglobin and plasma renin levels. At puberty, white male children have decreased high-density lipoprotein (HDL) levels and increased low-density lipoprotein/HDL ratios. Black children have lower urinary K excretion. Rational approaches to primary prevention of arteriosclerosis and hypertension may require a diversity of strategies because of these black-white differences.

3. Blumenstein, B.A., Douglas, M.D. and Hall, W.D. "Blood Pressure Changes and Oral Contraceptive Use: A Study of 2676 Black Women in the Southeastern United States." American Journal of Epidemiology 112 (4) (October 1980): 539-52.

Blood pressure (BP) and weight were measured on 2676 black women attending a large southeastern family planning clinic. Repeat measurements were made after a minimum of six and up to 24 months on 673 new women who continuously used nonhormonal contraceptive (OC) therapy, and 1390 women who had continuously used OCs. The mean change in systolic blood pressure (SBP) adjusted for initial BP and change in percent ideal body weight is +1.44 mm Hg in the new users of OC. This slight increase in SBP is statistically significant (p = 0.04) relative to the +0.41 mmHg increase observed in the control group. However, the adjusted diastolic blood pressure (DBP) change (+0.46 mmHg in new OC users and +1.54 mmHg in the control group) fails to support the hypothesis of a greater increase in DBP in new OC users. The adjusted mean rise in mean arterial BP does not differ significantly between new OC users and the control group. The mmHg during the average follow-up interval of one year is 2.4% in the control group, 1.0% in the new OC users and 0.2% in the continued OC users. These results provide evidence that OC use has no significant effect on the level of mean arterial BP in black women followed for 6-24 months; and fail to support the hypothesis of a causal relationship between OC use and elevated BP in black women.

4. Connett, J.E. and Stamler, J. "Responses of Black and White Males to the Special Intervention Program of the Multiple Risk Factor Intervention Trial." American Heart Journal 108 (3) (1984): 839-48.

Of the 12,866 males age 35 to 57 years who were randomly assigned to the Multiple Risk Factor Intervention Trial, 931 (7.2%) were black. All were assessed to be in the upper 10% to 15% of coronary risk because of their diastolic blood pressure, serum cholesterol level, and/or cigarette use. Attendance rates over the years of the trial were similarly high for blacks and whites. Smoking cessation rates, changes in dietary lipid composition and in plasma total and cholesterol, and achievement of normotensive diastolic pressure were comparable for black and white males. This experience indicates ability to induce extensive changes in lifestyles of both black and white American males.

5. Cruckshank, J.K. "Epidemiology and Hypertension: Blood Pressure in Blacks and Whites." Clinical Science 62 (1) (January 1982): 1-6.

There are genuine differences between races concerning blood pressure. Different social classes may also account for different levels of blood pressure and mortality. Good control of blood pressure leads to prevention of death from heart attacks and stroke in both blacks and whites. Higher mortality of blacks may be due in part to less reliable medical care and reduced compliance with drug therapy. When blacks received medical care comparable with that of their white peers, their blood pressures and mortality fell.

6. Curry, C.L., Oliver, J. and Mumtax, F.B. "Coronary Artery Disease in Blacks: Risk Factors." American Heart Journal 108 (3) (Part 2) (September 1984): 653-57.

The current literature indicates that of the major risk factors for coronary artery disease (CAD), United States blacks and whites have similar rates for cigarette smoking and cholesterol levels. The prevalence of diabetes mellitus is higher in black females than white females. Both black males and females have higher prevalence rates for hypertension. These differences in risk factors between blacks and whites in spite of similar degrees of CAD suggest that the relative importance of specific risk factors might differ between the two racial groups. Research is needed to determine if there are protective factors in blacks (e.g., high-density lipoprotein cholesterol) and/or previously unrecognized risk factors (e.g., diuretic-induced lipid abnormalities) that may be playing a major role in the epidemiology of CAD in the black population.

7. Garfinkel, L. "Cigarette Smoking and Coronary Heart Disease in Blacks: Comparison to Whites in a Prospective Study." American Heart Journal 108 (3) (1984): 802-7.

The American Cancer Society's prospective study of 1 million Americans was analyzed to determine whether coronary heart disease (CHD) mortality rates by cigarette smoking in blacks differed from those in Whites. More than 22,000 blacks were followed up for nearly 200,000 person-years in the 12-year study, 1960-1972. A total of 642 black males and 487 black females who died of CHD at age 40 and older were included. CHD mortality ratios by number of cigarettes smoked were about the same at given smoking levels in black and white males and were slightly lower in black than in white females.

8. Gartside, P.S. et.al. "Determinants of High-Density Lipoprotein Cholesterol in Blacks and Whites: The Second National Health and Nutrition Examination Survey." American Heart Journal 108 (3) (1984): 641-53.

Using 19,521 subjects (8259 and 8561 white males and females; 1299 and 1402 black males and females) in the second National Health and Nutrition Examination Survey, the study assesses black-white differences as major determinants of high-density lipoprotein (HDL) cholesterol to determine whether higher levels of HDL cholesterol in blacks can be accounted for by black-white differences in nutrient intake, relative ponderosity, alcohol intake, cigarette smoking, leisure-time and habitual physical activity, hypertension, and diabetes.

9. Gillum, R.F. and Gillum, B.S. <u>Potential for Control and Prevention of Essential Hypertension in the Black Community Behavioral Health: A Handbook of Health Enhancement and Disease Prevention</u> (N.Y.: John Wiley and Sons, 1984).

Blood pressure levels at any given age among black adults average 5 to 10 mm higher than those among white adults. Although it is uncertain whether genetic or physiological bases exist for these differences, the lower socioeconomic status and higher socioecological stress levels of blacks are probably important. Most surveys have found no consistent blood pressure differences between black and white children below the age of 10. The blood pressure differences seen in adults first become consistently apparent in adolescence. It is also interesting that blood pressures of blacks in America are consistently higher than even those of urbanized blacks in West Africa. The vascular sequelae of hypertension are the leading killers of blacks in the United States. For hypertensive disease and stroke the black-to-white mortality ratios are as high as 7 to 1, especially in younger age groups. This mortality is out of proportion to hypertension prevalence and is a reflection of inadequate hypertension detection and treatment. Black men have coronary heart disease rates similar to those of white men, but black women have much higher coronary heart disease rates than white women. This observation requires intensive investigation.

10. Gillum, R.F. and Kuller, L. "Coronary Heart Disease in Blacks: Myth versus Fact." <u>Urban Health</u> 13 (August 1984) 28-29.

Observes that there is a significant widespread opinion that coronary disease does not commonly affect blacks in the U.S. Refutes four myths which the authors argue "adversely affect the diagnostic and therapeutic care offered to the large number of black patients who present symptoms of coronary heart disease (CHD)." These myths are 1) CHD is uncommon in blacks; 2) blacks rarely have myocardial infarction or agina pectoris; 3) blacks have much less CHD than whites in the U.S.; and 4) blacks are immune to CHD. Argue that clinicians caring for black patients must become more aware and informed about CHD in the black community and that arteriosclerosis researchers should review, revise and/or offer new hypothesis on CHD in blacks.

11. Gluek, C.J. et.al. "High Density Lipoprotein Cholesterol in Blacks and Whites: Potential Ramifications for Coronary Heart

Disease." American Heart Journal 108 (3) (1984): 815-26.

Black male and female juveniles and adult black males have higher levels of high-density lipoprotein (HDL) cholesterol than do whites, differences that potentially "protect" them against augmented coronary heart disease morbidity and mortality, given an excess of certain coronary heart disease risk factors among blacks, particularly hypertension. The loss of the "protective" HDL cholesterol difference in adult black females appears most likely to be due to their pandemic obesity. It seems likely that whereas environment has a substantial effect on HDL cholesterol for blacks and whites, there may be a "genetic" vector accounting for higher levels of HDL cholesterol in blacks.

12. Haigh, N.Z. et.al. "The East Baltimore Study: The Relationship of Lipids and Lipoproteins to Selected Cardiovascular Risk Factors in an Inner City Black Adult Population." The American Journal of Clinical Nutrition 38 (2) (1983): 320-26.

Low socioeconomic status, inner city black adults, aged 20 to 40 years (24 males and 45 females) were randomly selected from East Baltimore, Maryland to study plasma lipid and lipoprotein levels. Several factors known to affect these levels also were examined: dietary intake, alcohol intake, degree of obesity (measured by body mass index), physical activity level, smoking, and hormone use. Compared to women, the men consumed more calories and more cholesterol; the men also had a lower body mass index than the women. None of the factors studied explained the relatively low total cholesterol and low density lipoprotein cholesterol levels in the inner city black adult men.

13. Harburg, E. et.al. "Skin Color, Ethnicity, and Blood Pressure I: Detroit Blacks." American Journal of Public Health 68 (December 1978): 1177-83.

Ranks census areas in Detroit for their stress scores based on instability and socioeconomic status. Four areas were selected for study: high stress, population predominantly black and white; low stress, population predominantly black and white. A sample was drawn from each area of persons of the predominant race, 25-60 years old, married and living with spouse, and having relatives living in the Detroit area. Three blood pressure readings were taken and skin color was rated. Results show that darker skin color, especially for black males, is related to higher blood pressure. Younger black males (25-39) in high stress areas had a higher pressure than males in low stress areas, regardless of skin color and weight. For older black males (40-59) darker skin color was correlated with higher blood pressure, regardless of weight or stress area. These findings suggest that varied gene mixtures may be related to blood pressure levels and that skin color combines with socially induced stress to induce higher blood pressures in lower class blacks.

14. Haywood, L.J. "Issues in the Natural History and Treatment of Coronary Heart Disease in Black Populations: Medical Management." American Heart Journal 108 (3) (1984): 683-89.

Data from multiple sources indicate that the death rate for blacks is higher than for the general population--in part because of higher mortality from cardiovascular causes. The Cardiovascular Mortality Survey, carried out in Los Angeles, indicates that the combined effects of increased mortality from high blood pressure and related causes, together with an ischemic heart disease mortality rate that is only a little below the mean, account for the overall excess mortality rates in blacks. In addition, black patients have been shown to have higher risk profiles compared with the study mean in a large study of beta-blocker therapy. Further studies of responses to therapy are suggested.

15. Haywood, L.J. "Coronary Heart Disease Mortality/ Morbidity and Risk in Blacks. II: Access to Medical Care." American Heart Journal 108 (3) (1984): 794-96.

Since the cardiovascular disease mortality is higher, life expectancy shorter, and socioeconomic conditions lower for black persons compared to the majority population, speculation arises as to the possible role of distribution of health resources for this segment of the population. Data from the City of Los Angeles, collected by health districts, confirm that deaths caused by ischemic heart disease occur at a lower age in blacks and that a dramatic fall in these rates (which are lower than for the majority population) has not occurred during the 1970-1979 period. Observations on some relevant factors and suggestions for further monitoring of health care needs and resources are offered.

16. Hosten, A.O. "Hypertension in Black and Other Populations: Environmental Factors and Approaches to Management." Journal of the National Medical Association 72 (2) (February 1980): III-17.

Hypertension is a major health problem for industrialized as well as developing countries, especially those with sizable black populations. Analyzes various aspects of hypertension in black and other populations with emphasis on contributing factors and therapeutic approaches. The facts seem to suggest that there is no intrinsic ethnic immunity to hypertension. Given a baseline genetic predisposition, a factor with which black people seem heavily endowed, superimposed with the right mix of environmental influences one might expect hypertension to be prominent. Therefore, no developing society, least of all one with a black heritage, should feel secure against this potential killer.

17. James, S.A. "Coronary Heart Disease in Black Americans: Suggestions for Research on Psychosocial Factors." American Heart Journal 108 (3) (1984): 833-838.

Despite the fact that coronary heart disease (CHD) is the leading cause of death among U.S. blacks, virtually no information exists on the contribution of psychosocial factors to CHD risk in this population. Studies conducted on U.S. whites suggest that type A behavior may be positively associated with risk for CHD. Other studies on whites suggest that occupational stresses, socioeconomic status, and social mobility may also be important. Studies that examine the contribution of these factors to CHD risk in the black population are needed. Some of the theoretical and measurement issues that investigators may face in conducting such research are discussed and some specific suggestions for research are offered.

18. James, S.A. et.al. "the Edgecombe County (NC) High Blood Pressure Control Program: Barriers to the Use of Medical Care Among Hypertensives." American Journal of Public Health 74 (5) (May 1984): 468-72.

As the initial step in a five-year project to improve control of high blood pressure in Edgecombe County, North Carolina, a survey was conducted in 1980 to determine the prevalence of hypertension and to identify factors which might constitute barriers to the use of medical care by hypertensives. This report summarizes the findings for the 539 hypertensives identified through the baseline survey. In general, black hypertensives reported more access problems than whites. Within race, however, males and females differed very little on selected measures of potential access to medical care. Among women, lower scores on potential access were strongly associated with being untreated, whereas for men, concerns about the safety of anti-hypertensive drug therapy were associated with being unaware. On a summary measure of the actual use of medical care in response to symptoms, both male and female treated hypertensives scored higher than their untreated counterparts. The implications of these and other findings for community based blood pressure control activities are discussed.

19. Karp, R.J. et.al. "Increased Utilization of Salty Food With Age Among Preteenage Black Girls." Journal of the National Medical Association 72 (3) (March 1980): 197-200.

In a survey of black inner-city school children 10 to 13 years of age, a significant correlation was found for obesity and systolic blood pressure. Significant correlation was found for obesity of mothers and daughters. No such relationships were found for mothers and sons. There was an increased consumption of sodium-rich foods by girls as their age increased, which was not found for boys. Both obesity and a sodium-rich diet are risk factors for the development of hypertension. The study suggests that among overweight black girls in the preteen years attempts should be made to limit consumption of salty foods and thereby limit weight gain.

20. Keil, J.E. et.al. "Incidence of Coronary Heart Disease in Blacks in Charleston, South Carolina." American Heart Journal 108 (3) (1984): 779-786.

A study of 2275 blacks and whites of both sexes in Charleston County, S.C., during the period 1960-1975. There were 317 new cases of coronary heart disease by 1975 in persons originally free of CHD. White males had the highest incidence rates. Black males and black females had the next highest rates. Angina pectoris in black females was double the rate in white females and five times the rate in white males. The rate of sudden death in black males was two and one-half times the rate in black females, three times the rate in white males, and four times the rate in white females.

21. Keith, T.A. "Renovascular Hypertension in Black Patients" Hypertension 4 (3) (May/June 1982): 438-43.

In a ten year period, 7200 of 19,000 black hypertensive adults in the University of Cincinnati Medical Center were referred to the Hypertension Service. In selected patients, intravenous urograms (1038) and renal arteriograms (238) were performed; 47 cases of renovascular hypertension (0.65% of the referred group and 0.25% of the entire sample) were identified. Atherosclerosis (32 patients) and fibromuscular dysplasia (11) were the most common causes of renal artery obstruction. Other lesions included traumatic thrombosis (1). Twenty-four patients were operated on (6 cured, 14 improved, 4 dead) and 23 treated medically (18 improved, 2 unimproved, 3 dead). Surgical mortality was 0. Follow-up exceeded 5 years in 25 patients. Extrarenal vascular lesions were found in 30 patients and accounted for six of seven deaths. Renal vein renin ratios greater than 1.5:1 (affected to unaffected side) predicted successful surgery in 14 patients, but eight of nine operated patients with ratios less than 1.5:1 also had favorable results. Factors in addition to renin assay were weighed before surgery was recommended. Since renovasuclar hypertension is rare in adult blacks, intensive investigation for this entity is justified only in patients with distinct suggestive findings. Treatment results in blacks are similar to those in white cohorts.

22. Kerr, G.R. et.al. "Ethnic Patterns of Salt Purchases in Houston, Texas." <u>American Journal of Epidemiology</u> 115 (6) (June 1982): 906-16.

Dietary sodium may play a contributory role in the development of hypertension, but difficulties in defining the "usual sodium intake of individuals prevent any stronger statement of the nature of the diet-disease relationship. The prevalence of hypertension is greater in black than in white populations of the United States, and there is speculation that dietary sodium intake may also be greater in black individuals. A significant proportion of dietary sodium is derived from table salt added to food during its preparation and consumption. In an attempt to identify whether purchase of table salt was sufficiently increased in black communities to support the hypothesis of an etiologic role in hypertension, the scales of table salt in supermarkets located in predominantly black, Hispanic and white census tracts of Houston, Texas, were compared. The mean ratio between sales of salt and a series of 20 staple food commodities in predominantly black and Hispanic census tract supermarkets were 148% and 202%, respectively, of that in predominantly white census tracts. The elevated ratios were not due to reduced sales of the food commodities. The authors conclude that sales of table salt, in relation to the series of food commodities, are 50-100% higher in Houston's black and Hispanic census tract supermarkets than in those of white census tracts. Whether the increased sales of table salt have causal relationship to the prevalence of hypertension in these communities can only be determined by further studies.

23. Kong, B.W. et.al. "Churches as High Blood Pressure Control Centers." <u>Journal of the National Medical Association</u> 74 (9) (September 1982): 920-23.

High blood pressure, a severe medical problem in the black community, can be controlled to a significant degree by proper medication. Discovery of hypertension and continuing therapy, however, are difficult. The establishment of churches as high blood pressure control centers is a promising approach to overcome these deficits. The initial experiences with the creation of such a program are presented. Difficulties include community unawareness of the seriousness of the problem, reluctance of volunteer workers to assume screening responsibility, reluctance of health professionals to accept the role of lay workers, and lack of technical proficiency in volunteers.

24. Heymsfield, S. et.al. "Race, Education and Prevalence of Hypertension." American Journal of Epidemiology 106 (5) (November 1977): 351-61.

Data from the Hypertension Detection and Follow-up Program (HDFP) in 14 U.S. communities were used to examine the relationship of education to the well-documented racial differences in prevalence of hypertension. Standardized blood pressure (BP) measurements, a medical history, and socioeconomic information were obtained on 158,906 adults. Hypertensive individuals were defined as 1) those with a diastolic BP greater than or equal to 95 mm Hg and 2) those with a diastolic BP less than 95 mm Hg who reported they were currently taking antihypertensive medication. Overall, 18.0% of whites and 37.4% of blacks were defined as hypertensive at the first screening. Education was found to be inversely associated with hypertension for each race and sex group. This inverse association remained when age was taken into account, was more striking in the younger age group and in blacks, but was diminished in the highest weight classes. Educational differences, however, do not fully account for the observed black-white differences in hypertension prevalence. Even at the higher education levels, the adjusted prevalence of hypertension remained nearly twice as high in blacks as in whites.

25. Langford, H.G. et.al. "Black-White Comparison of Indices of Coronary Heart Disease and Myocardial Infarction in the Stepped-Care Cohort of the Hypertension Detection and Follow-Up Program." American Heart Journal 108 (3) (Part 2) (September 1984): 797-801.

As part of the initial examination of individuals enrolled in the Hypertension Detection and Follow-Up Program, a standardized questionnaire to elicit symptoms of angina pectoris and myocardial infarction and to inquire about the clinical diagnosis of myocardial infarction was administered. Angina pectoris was more prevalent in black males than white males and more prevalent in black females than white females. In white and black males and in white females, baseline prevalence of angina was associated with an approximate doubling of the 5-year mortality. A positive Rose Questionnaire for myocardial infarction, a positive clinical history of myocardial infarction, or a positive ECG for mortality was associated with increased mortality in all of the race-sex groups, with the exception of black females, in whom the ECG evidence of myocardial infarction at baseline was only modestly associated with mortality. The Rose Questionnaire evidence of myocardial infarction was actually associated with a lesser 5-year mortality. The higher prevalence of angina pectoris in black hypertensive males in the face of a high prevalence of hypertension in blacks suggests that the combination of coronary artery disease and hypertension is more of a health problem in black males than in white males. The situation in black females, however, is less clear. The 5-year incidence of myocardial infarction, positive ECG or history, or positive Rose Questionnaire was approximately equal in blacks and whites among the treated hypertensive patients.

26. Leaverton, P.E. et.al. "Coronary Heart Disease Mortality Rates in United States Blacks, 1968-1978: Interstate Variation." American Heart Journal 180 (3) (1984): 732-37.

Among white males and females, recent declines in mortality from coronary heart disease (CHD) have not been uniform by region or state. To describe trends for the black population by states, a comparison is made of CHD death rates for persons aged 35-74 years for the years 1969-1972 in combination with rates for 1978. Reported mortality from 34 states with reasonably large black populations is described. Not all of the recent geographic shifts for white CHD mortality rates were apparent for blacks. Yet there were similarities, notably a slower decline, and therefore, a worsening of relative CHD mortality in West Virginia and Kentucky.

27. Lewis, E.A. "High Blood Pressure, Other Risk Factors and Longevity: The Insurance Viewpoint." American Journal of Medicine 55 (September 1983): 281-94.

Points out that black men aged 45 to 65 with elevated systolic or diastolic blood pressures appear to be double that of white men. In black women aged 45 to 54, the proportion is about two and a half times that among white women. Among black women aged 55 to 64, the proportion is only about a third higher than among white women. High blood pressure in blacks seems to be related to their generally lower socieconomic status and also may be related to a genetic factor. This conclusion is based on observations that hypertension is quite common in West African tribes, whereas average blood pressures in several East African tribes resemble more nearly those of whites in the United States.

28. Lynds, B.G., Seyler, S.K. and Morgan, B.M. "The Relationship Between Elevated Blood Pressure and Obesity in Black Children." American Journal of Public Health 70 (2) (February 1980): 171-73.

Blood pressures, heights and weights were measured in 1,692 elementary school black children. Elevated blood pressure (EBP) was defined as a systolic or diastolic reading above the 90th percentile for age, and weights were categorized into five classes based on weight for height norms. Systolic EBP children, whether boys or girls, were three times as likely to be obese as black children in the total population, and a similar relationship held for diastolic EBP children.

29. "Minorities in Medical Schools 1968-78." Journal of Medical Education 53 (8) (August 1978): 694-5.

Addresses historic events and efforts to increase minority enrollment in medical schools from 1968. Looks at provisions for admission based on class structure prior to 1968 as key to admission. Addresses substantial increase by medical schools and organizations and individuals to increase participation of minorities during past 10 years.

30. Neaton, J.D. et.al. "Total and Cardiovascular Mortality in Relation to Cigarette Smoking, Serum Cholesterol Concentration, and Diastolic Blood Pressure Among Black and White Males Followed Up for Five Years." American Heart Journal 108 (3) (1984): 759-69.

The Multiple Risk Factor Intervention Trial screening program provided an opportunity to study the association of diastolic blood pressure level, serum cholesterol concentration, and cigarettes per day with mortality after 5 years among 23,490 black males and to compare these associations with those observed among 325,384 white males. Diastolic blood pressure was more positively associated with cerebrovascular disease deaths among black males than white males according to the analysis. These findings suggest that the causes of CHD and cerebrovasuclar disease may be different for black and white males, particularly in regard to how these disease processes relate to blood pressure.

31. Oberman, A. and Cutter, G. "Issues in the Natural History and Treatment of Coronary Heart Disease in Black Populations: Surgical Treatment." American Heart Journal 108 (3) (1984): 688-94.

Patient characteristics, treatment choices, and long-term survival were examined to seek possible explanations for marked differences in the racial distribution among 6594 consecutvie patients who underwent arteriography or coronary artery bypass grafting from 1970 to 1978. Overall, the percentage of whites undergoing coronary arteriography was 96% compared with 4% of the blacks; only black females showed an increase in the relative percentage. Except for older blacks, who demonstrated a decreased survival rate when managed surgically, survival rates were similar for blacks and whites. Trends in the evaluation and clinical management of black populations with suspect coronary heart disease should further clarify these preliminary findings.

32. Pierre, T. "The Relationship between Hypertension and Psycho-Social Functioning in

Young Black Men." Journal of Afro-American Issues 4 (Summer/Fall 1976): 408-19.

Examines relationship of psycho-social functioning to a diagnosis of hypertension among black men age 15 to 25. The largest category of hypertension falls under the heading "essential," which means that there is no known cause or curable form. Recent studies have provided evidence indicating a significant number of adolescents are diagnosed as hypertensive indicating that stress and frustration begin at an early age for black youths. Black youths between the ages of 15 to 25 who are hypertensive experience numerous frustrations. Hypertensive individuals also tend to internalize frustrations. Black American men have a predisposition to hypertension and stress and frustrations are an important component of that predisposition. In light of this information, we must begin to investigate teaching skills which allow and individual to cope with stress and frustrations.

33. Remingston, R.D. "High Blood Pressure Control: What Are the Next Steps?" Public Health Reports 95 (5) (September/October 1980): 456-61.

Steps need to be taken to alleviate high blood pressure in blacks and whites alike. Work needs community blood control efforts, to expand the frequency with which hypertension is detected, bring increased percentages of hypertension under pharmacological and nonpharmacological control, and expand the vigorous management of the blood pressure to achieve levels within the normal range. There is a general lack of understanding as to why there ia a two-fold increase in hypertension prevalence of U.S. blacks over U.S. whites.

34. Rowland, M.L. and Fulwood, R. "Coronary Heart Disease Factor Trends in Black Between the First and Second National Health and Nutrition Examination Surveys: United States, 1971-1980." American Heart Journal 108 (3) (Part 2) (September 1984): 771-79.

This article focuses on changes in prevalence of three of the major risk factors for coronary heart disease (CHD) among the black population age 25 to 74 years: blood pressure, cigarette smoking, and serum cholesterol. It also examines the extent to which changes in these risk factors might explain changes in observed CHD mortality. These national estimates of risk factor levels among the black U.S. population are based on cross-sectional data from the National Health and Nutrition Examination Surveys of 1971-1975 and 1976-1980. Results of analyses show that there was a large and statistically significant decrease in the prevalence of elevated blood pressure for black adults between the two time periods; there was a large, significant decrease in the percent of black females who smoke and a smaller decrease in the proportion of black males who smoke; and there was no statistically significant change in the prevalence of elevated serum cholesterol. In addition, the percent of black adults with two or more risk factors decreased between 1971-1975 and 1976-1980. Lower levels of the three risk factors appear to explain a portion of the decline in observed CHD mortality for blacks. However, despite the encouraging lower prevalence of risk factors for blacks, more than 60% of the black adults 25 to 74 years of age still had one or more CHD risk factors in 1976-1980.

35. Sterling, R.P. et.al. "Results of Myocardial Prevascularization in Black Males." American Heart Journal 108 (3) (1984): 695-99.

Because the impact of black-white differences in the prevalence of risk factors for coronary heart disease on the outcome of coronary bypass surgery has not been well defined, preoperative status, coronary anatomy, and surgical results were reviewed in 54 black males who underwent operations between December 1970 and August 1983. Although immediate operative mortality appears not to be affected by black-white status, long-term prognosis may be influenced significantly by the high prevalence of hypertension and diabetes and the lower prevalence of hyperlipidemia among black patients. The relative risk imposed by genetic, metabolic, and physiologic characteristics may be influenced by social and behavioral considerations, such as access to medical care and patient compliance.

36. Strong, J.P. et.al. "Coronary Heart Disease in Young Black and White Males in New Orleans: Community Pathology Study." American Heart Journal 108 (3) (1984): 747-59.

The biracial population of New Orleans has a high overall mortality rate, high coronary heart disease (CHD) mortality rate, and high autopsy rate. This study investigated arteriosclerosis and CHD in all deceased males aged 25 to 44 years. Morphologic correlates of CHD were the same in young black and white males. CHD mortality and mortality from cerebral hemorrhage, hypertensive heart disease, chronic renal disease, and diabetes were greater in young black males than young whites. CHD mortality and mortality from cerebral hemorrhage, hypertensive heart disease, chronic renal disease, and diabetes were greater in young black males than young white males. The extent of coronary lesions had decreased between 1960 and 1978 in young white males but not in blacks. Racial differences in coronary lesion involvement in non-CHD deaths were smaller than in earlier studies.

37. Tebben, M.P. "HHS Demonstration Projects for Hypertension Control Focus on Blacks and Hispanics." Public Health Reports 97 (1) (January/February 1982): 80.

The Department of Health and Human Services has awarded $500,000 for the establishment of demonstration projects for hypertension control at five sites serving predominantly black and Hispanic populations. The demonstration projects will implement recommendations of the Black Health Providers Task Force on Hypertension Education and Control, which recently completed an eighteen-month study of high blood pressure. Uncontrolled high blood pressure is the number one health problem for black Americans, affecting an estimated five million persons. Blacks in certain age groups have from three to four times the rate of fatal stroke found in the general population, and they also have higher rates of heart and kidney disease.

38. Tebben M.P. "Trilateral High Blood Pressure and Control Project Aimed at Black Americans" Public Health Reports 97 (4) (July/August 1982): 386

The Department of Health and Human Services entered into a two-year $200,000 contract with the American Red Cross to work with major black groups on the problem of hypertension among black Americans. The effort is called the Trilateral High Blood Pressure and Control Project and is a collaborative effort of the public, private, and volunteer sectors. In the project, appropriate hypertension education and control strategies will be identified. A national advisory work group, composed of prominent black physicians, lawyers, and community leaders with an interest in the problems of high blood pressure among blacks, will assist the Red Cross in fostering the involvement of voluntary, religious, professional, civic, and business group in high blood pressure education and control activities.

39. Wilson, P.W. et.al. "HDL-Cholesterol in a Sample of Black Adults: The Framingham Minority Study." Metabolism 32 (4) (April 1983): 328-32.

A group of 100 adult black residents of Framingham, MA were examined and their plasma lipids were determined by the Framingham Heart Study Lipoprotein Laboratory. The age range of the participants was 20-69 years, and the mean age was 42 years for both sexes. The mean plasma total cholesterol, HDL-cholesterol (HDL-C), and triglyceride (TG) values for the 45 black men were 184,37.2 and 78 mg/dl, respectively. The corresponding levels for the 55 black women were 192,50.4 and 49. Even after adjusting for obesity, alcohol intake and cigarette use, the HDL-C levels among blacks were significantly lower (p less than 0.0001) than the levels for

Framingham white men and women. This black sample is more highly educated than black groups previously studied and appears to be as active as the Framingham white sample. Concludes that this black population has quite low HDL-C levels, and the results suggest that the lipoprotein distributions in this group differ from those previously reported for blacks.

2. Mental Health

40. Adebimpe, V.R. "White Norms and Psychiatric Diagnosis of Black Patients." American Journal of Psychiatry 138 (3) (March 1981): 279-85.

   Allegations of psychiatric misdiagnosis of black patients are supported by only a few examples of such errors, but there is a modest body of circumstantial evidence suggesting that black patients run a higher risk of being misdiagnosed than white patients. It has been alleged that because of racism in psychiatry, black patients are overdiagnosed in some categories and underdiagnosed in others, and that a white psychiatrist may attach a different pathological significance to the same behavioral deviation in white patients. The author reviews studies providing such evidence and concludes that greater awareness among clinicians and research into more appropriate diagnostic criteria for black patients are desirable.

41. Adebimpe, V.R. et.al. "Symptomatology of Depression in Black and White Patients." Journal of the National Medical Association 74 (2) (February 1982): 185-90.

   Compares the symptoms of public mental patients diagnosed as having a depressive disorder and relates the findings to the previous literature concerning black-white differences in mental illness. Findings corroborate previous observations that a somewhat smaller proportion of black admissions than white admissions are diagnosed with a depressive disorder and that a higher proportion of black admissions are diagnosed with a schizophrenic disorder. Some black-white differences in depressive symptoms were also corroborated--notably, slightly higher percentages of hostility, dangerousness, and somatic complaints in blacks--and these appeared to be independent of socioeconomic status.

42. Adebimpe, V.R., Klein, H.E., and Fried, J. "Hallucinations and Delusions in Black Psychiatric Patients." Journal of the National Medical Association 73 (6) (1981): 517-20.

A higher incidence of hallucinations have been previously reported among blacks as compared to whites. In contrast to these reports, which relied on hospital records, this study utilized standardized research rating scales, and confirmed the above observation among schizophrenic patients. Some blacks, irrespective of diagnosis, probably experience a variety of non-schizophrenic hallucinations, which when observed by unwary clinicians, may lead to erroneous diagnoses of schizophrenia. Current ignorance regarding the content of hallucinations in normal and non-schizophrenic and in schizophrenic blacks is a source of diagnostic confusion which may have dire consequences for many individuals.

43. Ausubel, D.P. "The Role of Race and Social Class in the Psychiatric Disorders of Treated Narcotic Addicts." International Journal of Addictions 15 (2) (February 1980): 303-7.

To test a clinical impression that lower-class black narcotic addicts from a ghetto "welfare" setting primarily manifest reactive schizophrenia when they become mentally ill, whereas white lower-middle or working class addicts primarily manifest reactive depression when they become neurotic or psychotic. A series of 20 consecutive mentally ill addicts from each group were compared with respect to diagnosis. The two groups were matched for age and sex. The findings overwhelmingly supported the hypothesis and are interpreted as confirming it insofar as the nature of the two populations permitted. It was impossible, for example, to separate the effects of racial membership from those of social class or from an interaction between the two variables.

44. Baker, F.M. "Black Suicide Attempters in 1980: A Preventive Focus." General Hospital Psychiatry 6 (2) (April 1984): 131-37.

A retrospective chart review of black suicide attempters was completed to describe the sample in comparison to prior studies and to develop preventive strategies. This sample of 56 black suicide attempters was composed of 17 males and 39 females, a ratio of 1:2.3. Female attempters were younger, 54% had made a prior attempt and had a diagnosis of either affective illness (33%) or an adjustment reaction with depressive features (31%). Male attempters were older, 76% had a prior psychiatric history, and 59% had a psychotic diagnosis. The potential for life-threatening behavior in psychotic blackman patients was noted. The necessity of monitoring the access to medication by stressed impulsive youth was emphasized.

45. Barbara, O.A., Maish, K.A., and Shorter-Gooden, K. "Mental

Health Among Blacks: The Reference of Self-Esteem, Commitment to Social Change and Paradoxical Attributions" Institutional Racism and Community Competence. (Rockville, MD.: U.S. Government Printing Office, 1982): 114-124.

Models of positive mental health are reviewed and assessed with respect to their applicability to blacks. A high level of self-esteem and an internal locus of control were consistently described as critical dimensions of effective functioning. These two factors, along with commitment to social change, were examined in three related studies of positive mental health in blacks. Negligible racial differences in self-esteem helpers. Strategies to improve service delivery are suggested.

46. Bell, C.C. "Black Intrapsychic Survival Skills: Alteration of State of Consciousness." Journal of the National Medical Association 74 (10) (October 1982): 1017-20.

Presents the thesis that the ability to alter one's state of consciousness is in fact a survival skill useful in coping with the physiologic effects of stress. Discusses techniques indigenous to black culture for altering states of consciousness and offers phenomenologic transcultural evidence that black culture is quite sophisticated in the area of intrapsychic survival skills. Outlines some of the sources of stress on blacks, discusses the mastery of stress, and focuses on some methods blacks use to alter their states of consciousness to master the stress they face daily and avoid "survival fatigue."

47. Bell, C.C. and Mehta, H. "The Misdiagnosis of Black Patients with Manic Depressive Illness." Journal of the National Medical Association 72 (2) (February 1980): 141-45.

Argues that contrary to earlier beliefs blacks may well demonstrate similar prevalence rates for manic depressive illness when compared with whites. However, black manic depressive patients are frequently misdiagnosed as being chronic undifferent- iated schizophrenics and treated with major tranquilizers when lithium is the drug of choice. This contention is supported by three case histories and some institutional dynamics that cause this form of iatrogenic morbidity to continue to prey upon black psychiatric patients.

48. Bell C.C., and Mehta, H. "Misdiagnosis of Black Patients with Manic Depressive Illness: Second in a Series." Journal of the National Medical Association 73 (2) (February 1981): 101-7.

When compared to whites many black patients with manic depressive illness are frequently misdiag- nosed. In a survey of the outpatient psychiatric clinic at Jackson Park Hospital, findings show that black patients in this clinic have similar prevalence rates of manic depressive illness when compared to surveys of white patient populations. In addition, survey findings show that the demographic characteristics of this subgroup of manic depressive patients were very similar to those found in white manic depressive patients. Yet, when the past histories of these black manic depressive patients were reviewed, large numbers who were diagnosed as schizophrenic were not considered for treatment with lithium.

49. Bell C.C. et.al. "Prevalence of Isolated Sleep Paralysis in Black Subjects." Journal of the National Medical Association 76 (5) (May 1984): 501-7.

Presents the first survey to measure the incidence of sleep paralysis in a black population of healthy subjects and psychiatric patients. Suggests the possiblity that sleep paralysis indicates a difference in the neurobiology of whites and blacks should be proven and properly interpreted, as well as the possibility that sleep paralysis may indicate that blacks have more of these types of hallucinatory experiences than whites.

50. Boone, L.R. "The Black Executive: A Challenge for Psychiatry." Journal of the National Medical Association 74 (3) (March 1982): 245-49.

Observes that the task of developing a body of knowledge about specific problems, both intrapsychic and psychosocial, which influence a black executive's maturation, may be initiated. There is currently a definite interest among black executives in obtaining access to appropriate psychotherapeutic intervention. A psychotic graphical approach facilitates development of construct for analysis of and insight into transference phenomena that translate into organization based behavioral response to the black executive. Suggestions for therapeutic directions involved affective and thematic strategies, all contingent upon a productive, informed therapeutic effort. The therapeutic relationship is a most important element in treatment strategy with the black executive.

51. Bowser, B.P. "Racism and Mental Health: An Exploration of Racist's Illness and the Victim's Health." Institutional Racism and Community Competence. (Rockville, MD.: U.S. Government Printing Office, 1982): 107-11.

The field of mental health has had difficulty in developing an adequate conceptualization of racism as a mental health problem. The racist's dysfunctional thinking and behavior are discussed and placed within the current nosology of mental illness. In light of the pervasive and potentially devastating influence of racism, it is suprising that black rates of institutionalization are not higher than they are. The role of black community life, including the persistence of many "Africanisms", is explored as one explanation of the emotional resiliency of many blacks.

52. Bradshaw, W.H., "Training Psychiatrists on Working with Black in Basic Residency Programs." American Journal of Psychiatry (December 1978): 1520-24.

Recommends a method of integration of specific training for working with black and other minority patients in existing traditional residency programs. Additionally, discussion is conducted relative to psychotherapeutic issues and problems encountered in biracial therapy or transcultural therapy. Addresses program structure, the essential educational experience, clinical services and general principles involved in providing adequate care to minority patients.

53. Brantley, T. "Racism and It's Impact on Psychotherapy." American Journal of Pyschiatry 140 (12) (December 1983): 1605-8.

Discusses the need for dealing with racial differences in therapy. Not doing this has resulted in patients terminating treatment because they perceive therapists do not understand them as patients and individuals. Identifies the need for development of a definite concern for racial issues in any therapeutic encounter which relates to problems of racial prejudices and discrimination.

54. Bush, James A., "Suicide and Blacks: A Conceptual Framework." Suicide and Life Threatening Behavior 9 (4) (1976): 216-22.

A conceptual framework for studying suicide among black Americans as a youth phenomenon with rates between sexes relatively equal is proposed, including extragroup pressure. Framework is extended into the area of mental health planning and into behavioral science practice, highlighting the lack of research on suicide and current explanations. Hypotheses discussed include frustration/aggression, cultural shock, and family emaciation. The conceptual model predicts dangerous reaction levels among individual blacks when highly negative pressure and extragroup pressure cause a growing sense of worthlessness, inadequacy, and impotence. It is suggested that a transcendent character can be facilitated by agreement between the values of black and their intragroup (family friends, personal relations) in resistance to the pressures of the extragroup (work, interest, finances). The perspective is especially recommended for designing mental health policies and programs to reinforce and contribute to the well-being of predominantly black communities.

55. Cannon, M.S. and Locke, B.Z. "Being Black is Detrimental to One's Mental

Health: Myth or Reality? *Phylon* 38 (4) (December 1977): 408-28.

The relationship between race and mental health can be determined by assessing the success of the mental health movement in closing the gap between services to whites and blacks. Factors which have an effect on black mental health include underemployment, poor housing, disrupted families, lower education, and stressful life conditions. Terminology referring to white and black mental health phenomena must be standardized to make comparison possible. Melanin in black skin is not the cause of black-white mental health differentials. Blacks experience greater feelings of failure, more denial of respect and less opportunity for dignity. The poor are more likely to receive inferior health care, less experienced doctors, assignment to outpatient clinics, and more drug therapy with little psychiatric support treatment. The needed reorienting of mental health programs requires that traditional individualistic methods of treatment be replaced with methods sensitive to the social problems of specific groups. Recent data-gathering methods are conducive to this but not enough is being done. Black attitudes toward white researchers can be changed by altering the aims of research from the search for "black pathology" to developing understanding for the black social condition. The use of black researchers would aid in such an understanding.

56. Carroll, J.R. et.al., "Personality Similarities and Differences in Four Diagnostic Groups of Women and Drug Addicts." *Journal of Studies on Alcohol* 42 (5) (May 1981): 432-40.

Scores on the Personality Research Form (PRF) indicated more similarities than differences in the personalities of four diagnostic groups of women alcoholics and drug addict but significant difference in the personalities of whites and blacks. The women's PRF scores suggest that black alcoholics and drug addicts were generally more fearful, vigilant, self-protective and anxious to avoid pain, more belligerent, argumentative and threatening and had a greater need to control, influence and act forcefully than did their white counterparts. Black women also gave evidence of a greater need for structure and absolute standards and rules in an environment than did white women. It is possible that the black women studied were more sensitive to their environment than their white counterparts because in a society that has yet to achieve racial equality and harmony heightened vigilance may have survival value for members of a minority group.

57. Carter, J.H. "The Black Aged: Implications for Mental Health Care." *Journal of the*

American Geriatrics Society 30 (1) (January 1982): 67-70.

> Some of the problems associated with providing quality mental health care for aged blacks are discussed. It is postulated that treatment should be used selectively, not in terms of simplistic formulas or part-truths about aged blacks, but on the bases of clinical indications in differential diagnosis. The essence of improved mental health for blacks, regardless of sex or age, entails an unrelenting struggle by mental health professionals toward the removal of all vestiges of racism.

58. Carter, J.H. "Psychiatry, Racism and Aging." Journal of The American Geriatrics Society 20 (7) (July 1972): 343-46.

> Discusses the inadequacies in the treatment of aged black psychiatric patients and argues that training programs in psychiatry should include working with people of a different race. Notes that the philosophical and social aspects of black culture should receive more attention. Many black patients' psychiatric problems are related to race. For elderly blacks, there is a pressing need for better integration of mental health services with other health and social services. Concludes that the nation must eventually develop programs to make it possible for all Americans to cope, regardless of their race or age and that it is also time psychiatrists, in addition to looking at black pathology, review possibilities for relieving system deficiencies, including the impact of racism.

59. Carter, J.H. "Psychiatry's Insenstivity To Racism And Aging." Psychiatric Opinion (6) (December 1973): 21-25.

> Racism is clearly a mental health problem and places every black American in the position of being "psychologically terrorized, politically tyrannized, socially minimized and economically ignored." Because of racism mental health professionals have been guilty of making too many invalid generalizations about the black elderly, with too little selective research regarding the relevance of race to aging. What is acutally needed is a personal involvement in attacking racism which gives rise to most of the mental health problems of the black patient. The black, elderly psychiatric patient whose problems would be expected to be compounded by age constitutes a special group of patients who generally meet all of our current "accepted" criteria for treatment. Concludes that private practice of psychiatry, which typically treats the middle-class neurotic patient, is obviously more rewarding financially than service in public clinics or mental hospitals that treat the aged and severely mentally disturbed blacks.

60. Carter, J.H. "A Psychiatric Strategy For Aged Blacks In The Future." Proceedings Of Black Aged In The Future. Jacquelyne J. Jackson, Editor. (Durham, N.C.: Center For The Study of Aging And Human Development, Duke University, 1973): 94-100.

   Argues that within the past decade psychiatry has made only token efforts to combat racism and to improve psychiatric care for black patients, especially elderly blacks. Points out that in spite of preventive measures, anticipates that aged blacks in the future will be suffering some mental illness. Concludes that white therapists can be effective with black patients if they learn to understand the cultural and social values of blacks.

61. Carter, J.H. "The Black Aged: A Strategy for Future Mental Health Service." Journal of the American Geriatrics Society 26 (12) (December 1978): 553-56.

   Outlines sociological as well as psychological reasons for ethnicultural-based mental health and psychiatric care for blacks, particularly the black elderly. Explains that the differences in quality between the life experiences of whites and those of non-whites lead inexplicably to differences in the manifestations of black emotional problems. The psychiatric and emotional problems of blacks are linked with beliefs regarding illness, health, and institutionalized racism. The fact that mental hospitals are obviously lacking black patients indicates a lack of strategy and planning for the psychiatric care needs of elderly blacks. Mental health care planning and support should target psychiatric and psychological care programs designed to meet the actual and perceived needs of blacks.

62. Carter, J.H. "Alcoholism in Black Vietnam Veterans: Symptoms of Posttraumatic Stress Disorder." Journal of the National Medical Association 74 (7) (July 1982): 655-60.

   A definitive diagnosis of a posttraumatic stress disorder in black Vietnam veterans can be made when recognition is given not only to the stresses of war, but to racism. An aftermath of the war for black veterans has been an alarming increase in alcoholism, and uncontrollable rage. Two cases are described that are illustrative of the posttraumatic stress disorder and alcoholism in black Vietnam veterans. A brief discussion of salient issues that are crucial to diagnosis and treatment is presented.

63. Carter, J.H. and Green, P.D. "Black Services in Community Mental Health Centers: A Need for Technical Assistance." Journal of the National Medical Association 73 (5) (May 1981): 403-8.

   The experience of two black mental health professionals, who were invited to provide technical assistance to improve services to blacks in three community mental health centers in South Carolina are described. This was a new and unprecedented attempt to elucidate and correct the problems of inadequate mental health services for blacks, while improving compliance with affirmative action. Camouflaged in elite professionalism were subtle hostile feelings and negative beliefs about blacks. Despite improvements in the mental health systems of our nation, there are millions who remain unserved, underserved, or inappropriately served.

64. Collins, J.L. et.al. "Frequency of Schizophrenia and Depression in a Black Inpatient Population." Journal of the National Medical Association 72 (9) (September 1980): 851-56.

A retrospective study covering the period 1974-1978 was conducted on the inpatient population at the Department of Psychiatry, Howard University Hospital, for the two major diagnostic categories, major affective disorders (MAD) and the schizophrenias. Among the schizophrenias, the diagnoses of schizophrenia, paranoid type and schizophrenia, not otherwise specified, account for approximately 73 per cent of all schizophrenic diagnoses. The distribution of diagnoses among the MAD category demonstrated that approximately 74 percent of all diagnoses were accounted for by the subcategory depressive neurosis. The implications of these analysis conducted on all black patient populations who were diagnosed by non-white diagnosticians are discussed.

65. Cowan, M.A. et.al. "Level of Education, Diagnosis and Race Related Differences in MMPI Performance." Journal of Clinical Psychology 31 (3) (July 1975): 442-4.

MMPIs were obtained from eight groups of black and white, schizophrenic and nonschizophrenic, and highly educated and poorly educated psychiatric patients. Profiles were classified blindly by use of two rules (Sc greater than 70; Sc greater than PT). All but poorly educated blacks were classified correctly beyond a chance level. Almost half of the poorly educated black nonschizophrenics were misclassified as schizophrenic. Implications for diagnostic work are discussed.

66. Craig, T.J. and Huffine, C.L. "Correlates of Patient Attendance in an Inner-City Mental Health Clinic." American Journal of Psychiatry 133 (1) (January 1976): 61-65.

Of 140 patients seen at a psychiatric clinic serving a predominantly black, low-income population, 65% attended for four or more visits. Patients over age 30 and those with a diagnosis of psychosis or personality disorder remained in therapy for significantly longer periods than the rest of the group. Failure to prescribe medication was associated with early dropout, but this effect seemed to be attenuated with duration of therapy. The race of the patients and therapists did not seen to influence continuation in treatment, but such an influence may have been masked by differences in the therapists' experience.

67. Craig, T.J. "Racial Patterns In Liaison Psychiatry." Journal of the National Medical Association 74 (12) (December 1982): 1211-15.

A study of 362 consecutive referrals from the general medical and surgical wards of a university hospital serving a large nonwhite community revealed an association between provisions of active liaison and a higher rate of referral for whites than non-whites. Once referral was made, however, there was no evidence of substantial bias in the consultation process with regard to reason for referral, diagnosis, or recommendations.

68. Davis, W.E. and Jones, M.H. "Negro Versus Caucasian Psychological Test Performance Revisited" Journal of Consulting and Clinical Psychology 42 (5) (October 1974): 675-79.

Differences in proportion of Negroes versus Caucasians receiving schizophrenic, alcoholic, and depressive psychiatric diagnoses were found. Race, education (12 years or more versus 11 years or less), and diagnosis (schizophrenic versus nonschizophrenic were varied. Contrary to the results of past research, significant race-related main effects were found on the nine MMPI (Minnesota Multiphasic Personality Inventory) clinical scales Schizophrenics scored high on MMPI Pa and Sc, and poorly educated patients scored higher on Sc. Higher PA and SC scale scores were obtained from poorly educated Negroes but not from higher educated Negroes or Caucasians at both educational levels. The results are discussed in terms of education having an inculturating effect on minority groups and a selective process whereby poorly motivated minority group members drop out of school. More advanced education appears to have either a masking or obliterating effect on culturally determined differences, at least in those who appear to be motivated to continue their education. Negroes who are "better" educated, that is have learned to cope with the demands of the Caucasian educational system, would demonstrate attitudes, opinions and values similar to Caucasians. Thus, it would appear that valid MMPIs may be obtained from Negroes and, perhaps, members of other minority groups who have been exposed to sufficient conventional education.

69. "Equity and The Psychiatric Care of The Black Patient." Journal of Nervous and Mental Disorder 168 (5) (May 1980): 279-86.

Discusses a comparison of treatment of black patients in a Northeastern industrial region in 1975 as compared with treatment existing in 1950. Identifies that black patients in 1975 compared to 1950 are utilizing exclusively state hospitals for inpatient care. Additionally, 1975 black patients are receiving outpatient services at regional community mental health centers which were non-existent in 1950. Notes the reduced amount of black clinicians except on non-professional levels, and applies a concept of equity to survey results to identify social issues of importance in evaluating the equity of pyschiatric care for black patients.

70. Faulker, A.O., Heisel, M.A. and Simms, P. "Life Strengths and Life Stresses: Exploration in the Measurement of the Mental Health of the Black Aged." American Journal of Orthopsychiatry 45 (1) (January 1975): 102-10.

Describes an attempt to understand the self-concept, social charactersistics, personal strengths, and frailties of a group of older black men and women in order to tailor mental health and social work services to their needs. Difficulties inherent in obtaining such information were minimized by a methodology that integrated the research and service aspects of the project. Results of the pilot study and service implications are discussed.

71. Flaherty, J.A. and Meagher, R. "Measuring Racial Bias in Inpatient Treatment." American Journal of Psychiatry 137 (6) (June 1980): 679-82.

In a retrospective chart audit of 66 black and 36 white male schizophrenic inpatients, the authors found that black patients spent less time in the hospital, obtained a lower privilege level, and were given more p.r.n. medication and were less likely to receive recreation therapy and occupational therapy. Seclusion and restraints were more likely to be used with black patients. The authors rule out the possibility of more severe pathology in the black patients by global rating of an additonal 15 white and 15 black patients. Concluding that there was racial bias, they attribute it to subtle stereotyping and the staff's greater familiarity with white patients. They suggest increased recruitment of black professionals and the inclusion of blacks in each treatment team.

72. Flaskerud, J.H. "Community Mental Health Nursing: Its Unique Role in the Delivery of Services to Ethnic Minorities." Perspectives in Psychiatric Care 20 (1) (January 1982): 37-43.

Community mental health nurses have a unique role to play in the delivery of mental health services to ethnic minorities. Among all mental health professionals in community settings, they, alone, bring a health generalist and public health background to the delivery of services. A background that prepares them to adapt their practice to meet the needs of ethnic minority clients.

73. Gary, L.E. "Correlates of Depressive Symptoms Among a Select Population of Black Men." American Journal of Public Health 75 (10) (October 1985): 1220-22.

This study was undertaken to provide information on the impact of demographic factors, stressful life events and socio-cultural patterns of depressive symptomatology among 142 noninstitutionalized black men. The findings indicate that age, family income, household size, employment status and conflict between the sexes were related to the presence of depressive symptoms. When controls were introduced, only family income and conflict between the sexes were correlates of depressive symptoms among black men in this study.

74. Gary, L.E. (ed.) Mental Health: A Challenge To The Black Community (Philadelphia: Dorrance & Co., 1978).

A collection of essays examining mental health issues in the black community.

75. Gibbs, J.T. "Use of Mental Health Services by Black Students at a Predominantly White University: A Three-Year Study." American Journal of Orthopsychiatry 45 (3) (April 1975): 430-45.

During three academic years, 87 black students were counseled at the mental health clinic of a private western university. Their pattern of clinic use was compared with that of white students, and differences and similarities delineated in presenting problems, symptoms syndromes, and duration and termination of treatment. Knowledge of these problems and patterns may aid mental health professionals as well as college counselors and administration in planning adequate support services for minority students.

76. Helzer, J.E. "Bipolar Affective Disorder in Black and White Men: A Comparison of Symptoms and Familial Illness." Archives of General Psychiatry 32 (9) (September 1975): 1140-43.

Eleven black and 19 white men with conditions diagnosed as manic-depressive disease, manic type were given a systematic psychiatric interview. In addition, as many of their first-degree relatives as could be contacted were also interviewed. Demographic, clinical, and family history variables were compared for the two races. With the exception of a greater preponderance of alcoholism in the paternal relatives of the black men, few differences were found between the two groups in terms of the variables studied. It was concluded that the clinical and familial expression of bipolar affective disorder is similar in the two races.

77. Jones, B.E. et.al. "Survey of Psychotherapy with Black Men" American Journal of Psychiatry 139 (9) (September 1982): 1174-77.

Analysis of a questionnaire survey regarding psychotherapy with black patients. Recieved usable responses from 51 black and 42 white psychiatrists. Nearly 100% of the black psychiatrists and 48% of the white psychiatrists were currently treating black patients. The black male patients were typically married and 31-40 years old, had technical or semiprofessional occupations and some college education, sought treatment for depression or work-related problems and remained in therapy for 13 weeks or more. Aggression/passivity was the most frequent unconscious conflict among the black males, developing new coping mechanisms was the most difficult treatment stage, and racism was often a causative factor in their pathology or was an expressed symptom.

78. Jones, B.E. et.al. "The Clinical Picture of Mania in Manic-Depressive Black Patients." Journal of the National Medical Association 74 (6) (June 1982): 553-57.

Argues that misdiagnosis of manic-depressive illness among blacks is a frequent occurrence. There are a number of historical and institutional dynamics involved which are attributed to racism. Examines the clinical symptoms and behaviors of manic-depressive illness among black patients to determine if their interpretation might be another contributing factor in misdiagnosis. Findings indicate that the clinical symptoms of manic-depressive illness in black patients be essentially what one would expect as determined by criteria in the Diagnostic and Statistical Manual. However, there were cultural and socioeconomic determinants of behavior that affected the clinical manifestations.

79. Jones, B.E. and Gray, B.A. "Black Males and Psychotherapy: Theoretical issues." American Journal of Psychotherapy 37 (1) (1983): 77-85.

The field of psychiatry has given insufficient attention to the issues of psychotherapy with blacks. Basic questions regarding what theories apply and what differences exist have seldom been addressed. The topic of black males and psychotherapy presents a multitude of theoretical questions. Only a few studies have attempted to address the relationship between the psychological problems of the black male and racism. As a result of racism, black males face internal and external obstacles that possibly cause psychic conflicts. This topic is reviewed from a theoretical perspective. Events that would precipitate black males' need for psychotherapy, where he would seek treatment, and conflicts presented in treatment are explored.

80. Jones, B.E. and Gray, B.A. "Similarities and Differences in Black Men and Women in Psychotherapy." Journal of the

National Medical Association 76 (1) (January 1984): 21-27.

A survey of 93 psychiatrists concerning the psychotherapy of black men and women indicated that there were more similarities than differences between the men and women. Black male patients age 31 to 40 and black women age 26 to 40 were most frequently seen for treatment. The patients were usually married and employed in technical or semiprofessional occupations. Both men and women had depression as the most frequent problem, with work related and family problems the next most frequent. For both the men and women, the psychiatrist felt racism was an important issue to consider in the treatment process and found that rage was related to racism.

81. Jones, B.E., Gray, B.A. and Parson, E.B. "Manic Depressive Illness Among Poor Urban Blacks." American Journal of Psychiatry 138 (5) (May 1981): 654-57.

In psychiatric epidemiology it has generally been accepted that manic-depressive illness rarely occurs among blacks and lower socioeconomic groups. The authors conducted a retrospective study to examine the frequency of manic-depressive illness among lower income urban blacks admitted to an acute psychiatric inpatient unit of an urban hospital. The medical records of a random sample of 117 black psychiatric patients were reviewed for determination of manic-depressive illness as well as socioeconomic characteristics. Eighteen subjects (15%) were diagnosed as manic-depressive. The authors present possible explanations for this finding and the ramifications for future investigations.

82. Jones E., "Social Class and Psychotherapy: A Critical Review of Research." Psychiatry 37 (4) (November 1974): 307-20.

Observes that persons from lower socioeconomic class backgrounds are less frequently accepted for treatment, are more likely to be assigned to inexperienced therapists and continue in therapy for a briefer period of time than their middle-class counterparts. Significantly more blacks than whites refuse treatment after an initial diagnosis.

83. Jones, W. "Preventing Mental Disorders in the Black Community: Approaches and Problems" Urban League Review 9 (2) (Winter) 1985/86): 32-38.

Examines a framework for preventive mental health in the black community. Programs for preventing drug abuse, alcohol abuse and mental illness among blacks must be enacted. Top priority must be given to program development, training, and research in primary prevention and emphasis should be directed to the youth of the community. An ultimate proactive preventive strategy might be to increase the power of blacks in society.

84. Kardiner, A. "Explorations in Negro Personality" in Culture and Mental Health, M.K. Opler (ed.) (New York: The Macmillan Company 1959): 413-24.

Argues that the ability to tolerate social inequities, such as slavery and social stratification, has been a significant factor in the role of Negroes throughout American history. The primary issue is that social discrimination affects individual personality. Although several features of Negro personality affirm social cohesion, such as the unity of feelings and opinions regarding Negro status in a white society, the discussion points to overwhelming indicators of non-cohesiveness among their culture. Primarily the result of having to identify with whites and with those characteristics in common with other American people whose culture and destiny they share. The social "fate" of the Negro is examined in light of such cohesiveness/lack-of-cohesiveness. Presents the theory that loss of pride in culture, the loss of male pride and the emerging superior role of the female in the Negro family are the three primary reasons for the breakdown of the Negro family. Thus impairing the ability for young blacks to cultivate emotions necessary for culture cohesion. Personality and culture breakdown theories are linked to mental health needs among Negroes.

85. Kasl, S.V. "Social and Psychological Factors in the Etiology of Coronary Heart Disease in Black Populations: An Exploration of Research Needs." American Heart Journal 108 (3) (1984): 660-69.

A number of findings that have broad relevance for the planning of future studies of psychosocial risk factors for coronary heart disease (CHD) in blacks are examined. These include data on marital status, social networks, health practices, well-being, distress, mental health, the residential environment, components of high blood pressure control, and health attitudes among youth. Conclusion suggests that the specific research literature on psychosocial risk factors for CHD is almost entirely based on the study of white populations and does not constitute a compelling basis for recommending research programs on blacks. It suggests a comprehensive examination of the psychosocial aspects of the black experience.

86. Keisling, R. "Underdiagnosis of Manic-depressive Illness in an Hospital Unit." American Journal of Psychiatry 138 (5) (May 1981): 672-73.

Examines whether blacks have a lower incidence of affective disorders. Findings support suggestions of Pope and Hispinski that manic-depressive illness is underdiagnosed in the U.S. No evidence was found that manic-depressive illness is less prevalent among blacks and minority groups as compared to whites.

87. Khaton, O.M. and Carriera, R.P. "An Attitude Study of Minority Group Adolescents Toward Mental Health." Journal of Youth and Adolescence 1 (2) (June 1972): 131-41.

An attitude study was conducted to ascertain the existence of any evident special attitudes towards mental health services as a result of being a part of a black or Spanish-speaking minority group. A total sample of 103 high school students at the junior and senior levels was chosen and a questionnaire was administered regarding the general area of mental health. The differences and similarities of responses were noted and recorded as they appeared, according to age, sex and subculture. Although specific group characteristics were revealed that might be soci-cultural such as student revolution, drug abuse, and changing sexual mores, the overall conclusion is that attitudes relating to the mental health field and its personnel are parallel to the majority population's beliefs. No evidence was found to support the contention that members of this population are not good insight patients, but rather it was found that insight is an individual capacity rather than a culturally determined one.

It is hoped that further research under more controlled conditions may provide conclusive evidence as to whether specific cultural attitudes do exist.

88. Koegel, P. and Edgerton, R.B. "Labeling and the Perception of Handicap Among Black Mildly Mentally Retarded Adults." American Journal of Mental Dificiency 87 (3) (November 1982): 266-76.

Participant observational research and interviewing with 45 black young adults who were labeled mildly mentally retarded during their school years indicated that the majority of these persons continued to label themselves in various ways and to perceive themselves as adaptively limited. Moreover, all of their parents labeled their adult children and recognized limitations in their adaptive behavior. Observations confirmed the presence of various adaptive limitations. Concludes that these black mildly retarded adults did not "disappear" into their communities but continued to see themselves and be seen by others as limited in adaptive skills, particularly "academic" skills such as reading and writing.

89. Lawson, W.B., Yesavage, J.A. and Werner, P.D. "Race, Violence, and Psychopathology." Journal of Clinical Psychiatry 45 (7) (July 1984): 294-97.

The frequency of violent behavior among inpatients in an acute psychiatric unit for veterans was examined. Violent behavior was assessed using a modified Lion scale in 93 white and 24 black consecutively admitted inpatients receiving a fixed dose of neuroleptic. Blacks were significantly less violent according to the Lion scale. Item analysis revealed that whites made more violent threats, committed more violent acts against self, and were more likely to be secluded or restrained. Blacks were less likely to commit multiple acts against others, although the actual numbers of violent episodes were not significantly different. No racial differences were seen in serum neuroleptic level, psychopathology as measured by the BPRS, or admission status. The same racial differences in violence were seen when either schizophrenics alone or paranoid schizophrenics were considered.

90. Lewis, D.O., Balla, D.A. and Shanok, S.S. "Some Evidence of Race Bias in the Diagnosis and Treatment of the Juvenile Offender." American Journal of Orthopsychiatry 49 (1) (January 1979): 53-61.

Clinical and epidemiological evidence is presented indicating that many more black delinquent children and their families fail to receive needed psychiatric and medical services than do white delinquents. Explanations and implications of the reluctance or inability of white mental health professionals to diagnose serious psychopathology in the black delinquent population are explored.

91. Lightfoot, O.B. "Ethnic and Cultural Variations in the Care of the Aged. Psychiatric Intervention with Blacks: The Elderly - A Case in Point." Journal of Geriatric Psychiatry 15 (2) (1982): 209-13.

Discusses a range of issues confronting black Americans at different points in the life cycle. Special attention is focused on the black elderly. Black Americans, the black elderly among them, are a sizable group in this country with needs that approximate and parallel the needs of the majority, and needs that diverge and require more focused attention. It is hoped that this discussion can be listed as just one of many undertaken by this sponsoring group around this vital subject.

92. Lothstein, L.M. and Roback, H. "Black Female Transexuals and Schizophrenia: A Serendipitous Finding? Archives of Sexual Behavior 13 (4) (August 1984): 371-86.

While increasing numbers of individuals have identified themselves as transsexuals and requested sex reassignment surgery, the number of black female applicants is grossly underrepresented. Indeed, only 3% of the patients applying at the Case Western Reserve University (CWRU) Gender Identity Clinic (5 of 174 patients) were black females; and in one survey of nine gender identity clinics, only 1.1 of the applicants were black females. In this study, all five black female applicants who applied for transsexual evaluation to the CWRU Gender Identity Clinic served as subjects. The patients' characteristics, their psychological test results, clinical interview material, and psychological and psychiatric diagnoses are presented. All patients had severe psychopathology; three were schizophrenic, one was a schizophrenic character, and the last diagnosis as either a psychotic character or borderline personality. Among the hypotheses, it was suggested that black women may be "inoculated" against severe gender identity pathology and only exhibit such pathology as a consequence of a schizophrenic illness or severe bordeline schizophrenic state. The data also suggest that more attention should be placed on investigating the family and cultural dynamics related to transsexualism. The implications of these findings for developing a comprehensive theory of transsexualism are presented.

93. Lucas, F. "Miles to Go Before We Sleep" MH 59 (2) (Spring 1975): 14-16.

Much still needs to be done to move society toward more human treatment of the black woman's needs, and mental health professionals can play an important role in the process. Asks the question, "Are mental health professions meeting the needs of the Black woman?" Mental health professionals can assist in changing the stereotype and false images of black women through community education and action programs.

94. Luchins, D.J., et.al. "HLA-A2 Antigen in Schizophrenic Patients with Reversed Cerebral Asymmetry." British Journal of Psychiatry 138 (March 1981): 240-43.

The frequency of HLA-A2 was examined in 32 black and 22 white schizophrenic patients separated into two groups according to whether they had normal or reversed cerebral hemisphere asymmetries as determined by computed tomography. The black patients with reversed asymmetry had a significantly greater frequency of HLA-A2 as compared to black patients with normal asymmetry and a black normal control group. There were no significant differences for any other A, B, or C antigens. These findings also held when only the 22 black patients without evidence of brain atrophy were studied. The results for the white patients were in the same direction but did not reach statistical significance. These findings suggest that, at least for black schizophrenic patients, reversed cerebral asymmetry is associated with an increased frequency of HLA-A2.

95. Lyles, M.R. and Carter, J.H. "Myths and Strengths of the Black Family: A Historical and Sociological Contribution to Family Therapy." Journal of the National Medical Association 74 (11) (November 1982): 119-23.

The psychiatric evaluation and treatment of black Americans remains a source of difficulty for mental health professionals. Difficulties with treating blacks have prompted suggestions that psychiatric residency programs provide training in cultural issues in psychotherapy. In the past, a greater emphasis was placed on individual therapy than on the influence of racial and cultural factors on diagnosis and patient-therapist relationships. Examines the historical, sociological, an behavioral literature about black family life. Prevailing myths surrounding black families are contrasted with their seldom acknowledged strengths and adaptive behavioral patterns. This diverse scientific literature leads to specific implications for family therapy.

96. Mayo, Julia A. "Utilization of a Community Mental Health Center by Blacks: Admission to Inpatient Status." Journal of Nervous and Mental Disease 158 (3) (1974): 202-07.

The hypothesis that utilization of the community mental health center (CMHC) is influenced more by demographic and psychosocial characteristics of patients and by perceptions and values of purveyors of mental health resources than by availability and organization of services was verified. In the catchment area under study, blacks, the police, social agencies and the CHMC staff itself accepted and followed a traditional practice of blacks going to the city hospital. Findings were in the expected direction with regard to psychosocial characteristics. Blacks were more often perceived as having more symptoms/complaints of persecution, suspiciousness, drug and alcohol abuse, and seizures than the non-black patients. Clinical factors of diagnosis, treatment response or prognosis were of little relevance in differentiating black from non-black patients.

97. Mercer, K. "Black Communities' Experience of Psychiatric Services." International Journal of Social Psychiatry 30 (Spring 1984): 22-27.

Indicates a number of common and popular black responses to psychiatry by way of two pertinent questions: How do black people come to the attention of psychiatry? And secondly, what happens within the encounter?

98. Merritt, L. Black Ethnic Identity and Its Relationship to Mental Health Service Delivery Preference Choice. (Adelphi University, School of Social Work, 1977).

Addresses whether an ethnic frame of reference in the delivery of services makes a difference to black people, to what degree does it make a difference. The major hypothesis is that the stronger the degree of ethnic identity, the greater the preference for the more ethnically oriented service differences in preference choices between age groups and educational levels, but no differences for other demographic variables. The major hypothesis regarding degree of ethnicity and its relationship to preference for mental health service organization was substantiated by the data. The sub-hypothesis was substantiated except for age.

99. Mirowsky, J. and Ross, C.E. "Minority Status, Ethnic Culture and Distress: A Comparison of Blacks, Whites, Mexicans and Mexican Americans." American Journal of Sociology 86 (3) (November 1980): 479-95.

This study examines the psychological well-being of blacks, whites, Mexicans, and Mexican Americans. There are 2 perspectives on the differences in distress among these groups: the minority-status perspective and the ethnic-culture prespective. Within the context of the minority-status perspective, two hypotheses are tested: (1) Minority status per se is distressing. (2) Minority status is distressing only because it is associated with low social class. Within the ethnic-culture perspective, several additional hypotheses are tested.

100. Molica, R.F., Blum, J.D. and Redlich, F. "Equity and the Psychiatric Care of the Black Patient: 1950 to 1975," Journal of Nervous and Mental Disorders 168 (5) (May 1980): 279-86.

Examines the change/non-change of types, quality and quantity of mental health care in state hospitals in the northeast states from 1950 to 1975. The survey was a part of the Trends in Mental Health Project, a 25-year follow-up of the study conducted in 1950 by Hollingshead and Redlich entitled Social Class and Mental Illness (John Wiley & Sons, New York, 1958). In 1975, as compared to 1950, black patients were placed almost exclusively in state hospitals as opposed to private mental health facilities and state hospitals continued to provide most of the health services and programs utilized by black mental patients (in-patient care). In addition, there continued to be a definite lack of outpatient care (almost non-existent) for black patients, except for that provided by the regional community mental health center facilities. Outpatient care predominantly included only low intervention types of treatment and was provided by either semi- or non-professional staff. The survey results also indicate that black mental health care providers were almost non-existent at the professional level. The majority of blacks employed in the mental health profession were found in non-professional positions. The purpose of this comparison study is to discuss the continuing inequity present in mental health care, public and private, for black patients -- inpatient care, outpatient care, variety and methods of treatment, variety and types of programs available, and availability of any program manned by qualified mental health professionals. Policy development and issues for consideration in funding public health care programs are discussed with primary emphasis on cultural, ethnic, and ethical values between mental health care for Anglos versus non-whites.

101. Mukherjee, S. et.al., "Misdiagnosis of Schizophrenia in Bipolar Patients: A Multiethnic Comparison." American Journal of Psychiatry 140 (12) (December 1983): 1571-74.

The records of 76 bipolar (DSM-III) patients were reviewed for a history of previous misdiagnosis-- auditory hallucinations, early age at onset, and ethnicity. Ethnicity remained significantly associated with misdiagnosis of bipolar patients as schizophrenic even after all other significant variables were omitted. It appears from these data that black and Hispanic (Puerto Rican) bipolar patients may be at a higher risk than whites for misdiagnosis as schizophrenic, particularly if they are young and experience auditory hallucinations during affective episodes.

102. Munford, P.R. "A Comparison of the WISC WISC-R on Black Child Psychiatric Outpatients." Journal of Clinical Psychology 34 (4) (October 1978): 938-42.

The WISC and WISC-R tests are commonly used instruments in client evaluation and determine whether a child may be classified as "mentally retarded." The Weschler Scales were administered to 20 black child outpatients in this study with resulting test scores indicating the two to be essentially different with scores on the Verbal Performance and Full Scale IQ Subtests on the WISC-R significantly lower than those of the WISC. Order of administration was also found to be significant. Significancy was found when the WISC was given after the WISC-R but not if given before. The study indicates the tests to be highly correlated with the major implication that greater numbers of black children may be given developmental disability labels as a result of methodology and administration of the two tests.

103. Neighbors, H.W. "Professional Help Use Among Black Americans: Implications for Unmet Need." American Journal of Community Psychology 12 (5) (October 1984): 551-66.

Previous findings on black utilization have been largely obtained from racial comparison studies. Little attention has been paid to socio-demographic differences or the social psychological processes that affect help-seeking behavior within the black group. The present study analyzed data obtained from a national probability sample of the black population. A multi-dimensional contingency table analysis revealed that problems experienced by the lower income group were more serious than those experienced by the upper income group. Low-income respondents were also more likely to state that their personal distress was caused by a physical health problem. Income, however, was not related to the decision to seek professional help. The implications of these findings for understanding black illness behavior and the underutilization of services are discussed.

104. Newmark, C.S. et.al. "Racial Bias in an MMPI Index in Schizophrenia." British Journal of Clinical Psychology (September 1981): 215-16.

Racial bias was not evident in this study's sample. However, the number of black male schizophrenics incorrectly diagnosed approached statistical significance when compared with the number of white male schizophrenics incorrectly diagnosed. The need to cross-validate was obvious in this study.

105. Opler, M.K. "The Cultural Backgrounds of Mental Health" in Culture and Mental Health. M.K. Opler (ed.) (New York: The MacMillan Company 1959): 1-20.

Presents "etho-psychiatric" issues and theories outlining the effects of culture on mental health. Discusses identifying "paths to illnesses" associated with different cultures; different levels and approaches to treatment along class lines; role of culture in formulating a person's interpretations of experiences; and the influence of one's cultural and social backgrounds upon an individual's functioning are areas of major concern. Using a basically scientific research approach, the author seeks to legitimize a literary version of a "culture peronality study." The field of social psychiatry concerns itself with the impact of varying cultural and social environments upon human psychology. Mental health psychiatric services for minority or culturally-cohesive groups (Blacks, American Indians, Mexican-Americans) must address and dynamically overcome etho-psychiatric barriers and other inhibitors to patient treatment and utlization of services.

106. Parker, S. and Kleiner, R.J. Mental Illness in the Urban Negro Community (New York: The Free Press, 1966).

A study of 3,000 blacks which finds that mental illness was most likely to occur among those at the upper end of the socioeconomic scale who are upwardly mobile, and among those at the lower end of the scale who are downwardly mobile. The high rates in these two groups appear contradictory but are understood, the authors feel, when examined in context with the social-psychological variables of the study.

107. Payton, C.R. "Substance Abuse and Mental Health: Special Prevention Strategies Needed for Ethics of Color," Public Health Reports. (1) (January/ February 1981): 20-25.

> Substance abuse is very prevalent in minority communities. This abuse results in a delayed education, school non-attendance, and inevitable mental health problems. Not enough studies on substance abuse are done with respect to ethnicity. More studies are needed that would benefit minorities such as relevant statistics gathered and reported with respect to trends, attitudes, and drug use patterns of young people. Also, research that focuses primarily on charcteristics of the individual rather than on the social, psychological, and physical milieu in which the individual functions may result in distorted data. Measures of self-esteem, decision-making abilities, and other person-centered traits imply that the deviant behavior is the fault of the individual. Ethnics of color believe such behavior is too often caused by the political-social system.

108. Peck, D.L. "'Official Documenation' of the Black Suicide Experience." Journal of Death and Dying 14 (1) (1983): 21-31.

> Explores methodological limitations confronted by researchers who test theoretical statements using suicide data generated by public officials. A discussion of official reporting procedures observed in one medical examiner's office suggests that investigative standards for assessing equivocal death among blacks may be minimal in comparison to the more uniform evaluations and documentation of questionable death for whites. Data pertaining to socioeconomic characteristics, religious preference, and the influence of interpersonal and intrapersonal factors thought to impact upon the black victim's decision to engage in life-destructive behavior are reported and discussed. The findings suggest that the social worth criterion of the victim may influence the recording of suicide data. Suggestions are offered for increasing the reliability of official suicide data.

109. Pumariega, A.J. et.al. "Anorexia Nervosa in Black Adolescents." Journal of the American Academy of Child Psychiatry 23 (1) (1984): 111-14.

> The incidence of anorexia nervosa in black youth is believed to be extremely low to negligible.

Reports on two cases of adolescent black female patients, seen over a 6-month period, who developed anorexia nervosa. Literature on the epidemiology of this disorder is reviewed with special attention to references to blacks. Unique characteristics of the two patients and one other reported at length in the literature are also discussed, as well as questions about the possible rising incidence of this disorder among blacks and the perceived causes for this increase.

110. Raskin, A., Crood, T.H. and Herman, K.D. "Psychiatric History and Symptom Differences in Black and White Depressed Inpatients." Journal of Consulting and Clinical Psychology 43 (1) (February 1975): 73-80.

As a part of the larger National Institute of Mental Health multihospital, collaborative study of drug treatment in depression, 159 black patients were compared with 555 white patients on social, personality and psychiatric history variables, as well as presenting symptoms. In making these comparisons, race differences in age, social class status, and sex were controlled. Both black and white depressed patients were remarkably similar on presenting symptoms, especially the core symptoms of depression, when the groups were equated or controlled for age and social class differences. However, some differences did emerge on a number of hostility variables. There was a greater tendency toward negativism and the introjection of anger in blacks than in whites. In addition, depressed black males indicated that they were more likely than their white counterparts to strike back, either verbally or physically, when they felt their rights were being violated. There was also a very high incidence of suicide threats or attempts among black males.

111. Ridley, C.R. "Clinical Treatment of the Nondisclosing Black Client." American Psychologist 39 (11) (November 1984): 1234-44.

The clinical problem of the black client who is nondisclosing to the white therapist is examined. Individual verbal psychotherapy, which has its roots in Freud, often places the black client in a paradoxical situation. Although client self-disclosure is generally considered essential for maximizing therapeutic outcomes, complex intrapersonal, interpersonal and social factors often affect the black client's willngness to self-disclose. Regardless of the black client's level of self-disclosure, white therapist/black client relationships tend to result in unhealthful consequences for the client. Explores these consequences and concludes with two sets of recommendations to counteract the problem.

112. Rosenfield, S. "Race Differences in Involuntary

Hospitalization." Journal of Health and Social Behavior 25 (1) (March 1984): 14-23.

Central proposition is that the powerless or culturally marginal individuals are more severely reacted to for psychiatric disorders. Such individuals are more likely to be hospitalized for mental illness than are those in more powerful or conventional groups. Therefore, in terms of hospitalizations, they are more likely to experience a more coercive response of involuntary hospitalizations, as opposed to voluntary hospitalization. Study sample is approximately half white and half non- white and shows that with males and females combined, whites and nonwhites do not differ in the likelihood of hospitalization in general, type of hospitalization, or voluntary hospitalization per se. However, nonwhites are significantly more likely than whites to be involuntary hospitalized compared to all other dispositions. Analysis by sex show this difference is due to nonwhite males who are much more likely to be hospitalized involuntarily because they are more often brought into treatment by the police.

113. Roukema, R., et.al. "Bipolar Disorder in a Low Socioeconomic Population: Difficulties in Diagnosis." Journal of Nervous and Mental Disease 172 (2) (February 1984): 76-79.

The diagnosis of manic-depressive disorder, manic type, does not usually present a diagnostic problem when there is a clear history of the onset of symptoms. However, when the manic patient deteriorates and reaches the "end-state" of the illness, his symptoms may be similar to those of schizophrenia. This report describes three cases from a largely black, low socioeconomic population that were misdiagnosed as schizophrenic rather than as manic. Delay in seeking immediate treatment for early symptoms of mania is cited as the primary reason for these misdiagnoses. Also, other possible reasons are discussed.

114. Sager, C.J., Brayboy, T.L., and Waxenberg, B.R. Black Ghetto Family in Therapy: A Laboratory Experience (New York: Grove Press, Inc, 1970).

Examines many factors in caring for blacks in various aspects of health including mental health. Issues explored such as white therapists treating blacks who have a 300-year history of discrimination; black therapists and their ability to treat whites when viewed in the social and economic barrier contexts; and the role of therapists in treating families whose prime concerns are subsistence and survival. Notes that there are increasing difficulties for white middle-class therapists in treating "multiproblem" black families and that lower class patients, as a result of economics, seek treatment as a last resort. Due to failure on the part of white therapists in providing adequate health treatment and because the demeanor of clinic patients is changing as the black community becomes more militant, the authors state we need to examine how we view lower-class culture in general and poor black people in particular. Black patients often bring with them a history of abusive and humiliating contact with whites and this past is not left at the entrance to the health care facility.

115. Silber, T.J. "Anorexia Nervosa in Black Adolescents." Journal of the National Medical Association 76 (1) (January 1984): 29-32.

Anorexia nervosa has been considered rare or nonexistent among blacks. The reason for the selection of anorexia nervosa as the topic for this article was to alert practitioners to the new phenomenon of anorexia nervosa among black teenagers. A report of the presentation and clinical course of this disorder in two black female adolescents illustrates a serious medical psychiatric problem that may be increasingly detected among predisplayed teenagers of the black middle and professional classes. Unrecognized and incorrectly treated, the disease may run a fatal course in 20% of the cases. Differential diagnosis, etiology, and treatment of the conditon are reviewed.

116. Smith, A., Jr. "Religion and Mental Health Among Blacks." Journal of Religion and Health 20 (4) (1981): 264-87.

Examines the relationship between religion and black self-esteem and mental health. Religion is considered as one of the important retained black cultural traits, which continues to play a vital role in the mental health and survival strategies of Black Americans. Grier and Cobb's appraisal of the religion-mental health connection in black communities is examined, and different ways for mental health practitioners to think about religious phenomena and the primal partnership between religion and mental health are identified. Both religion and mental health can assume complimentary relationships and give critical perspective to the person or family seeking help. Both are challenged to help evaluate, diagnose, and transform the spiritual and moral malaise of our troubled time.

118. Smith, E.J. "Mental Health and Service Delivery Systems for Black Women," Journal of Black Studies 12 (2) (December 1981): 126-41.

Black women encounter a number of mental health related problems as a result of their racial, historical, cultural and structural positions in American society. The low income of black women subjects them to the stresses that often accompany poverty, malnutrition, psychosocial deprivation, and hypertension. Often this results in alcoholism or suicide. In both of these areas, black women are overrepresented. The author contends that to help black women through counseling, the therapist has to realize that poverty can be a leading factor in clients stress and mental illness. Therapists need to examine more thoroughly the life conditions and stresses of black women.

118. Smith, O.S. and Gundlach, R.H. "Group Therapy for Blacks in a Therapeutic Community." American Journal of Orthopsychiatry 44 (1) (1974): 26-36.

A program of group therapy aimed at grappling with the core problems of most blacks such as loss of self-identification and lack of projection of a productively healthy existence is described. The black experience is seen as akin to that of a control group in a laboratory experiment. Implications of decontrolling a control group in the even more rigidly defined setting of a therapeutic community are explored.

119. Steer, R.A. et.al. "Structure of Depression in Black Alcoholic Men" Psychological Reports 41 (3 pt. 2) (December 1977): 1235- 41.

The Beck Depression Inventory was self-administered to 103 black men receiving outpatient treatment for alcoholism, and scores were subjected to factor analysis using a maximum likelihood solution. Their meaningful oblique dimensions were identified as Cognitive-Affective Impairment, Retarded Depression, and Escapism. The factor structure of the black alcoholic men was descriptively compared to those previously reported for racially heterogenous patients. The factors of depression for the black alcoholic men were comparable to those described for the other clinical sample.

120. Steinberg, M.D. et.al. "Demographic and Clinical Characteristics of Black Psychiatric Patients in a Private General Hospital." Hospital and Community Psychiatry 28 (2) (February 1977): 128-32.

A study of 419 first admissions to a private general hospital psychiatric inpatient unit showed that only 8.8 per cent were blacks, while 23 percent of the population in the community were blacks. When compared to white patients, blacks were much less likely to be referred for hospitalization by private sources, were substantially younger, and had shorter hospitalizations. The most common diagnosis for blacks was paranoid schizophrenia. The authors conclude that despite the widespread availability of third-party insurance coverage, blacks use the private general hospital less often than whites and their patterns of use are substantially different.

121. Sue, S. et.al. "Delivery of Community Mental Health Services to Black and White Clients" Journal of Consulting and Clinical Psychology 42 (6) (December 1974): 794-801.

Comparisons were made of services rendered to 959 black and 11,904 white clients recently seen at 17 community mental health centers or facilities. Data collected included client's age, sex, income, education, marital status, diagnosis, assignment to type of treatment program, major services received, number of contacts, and assignment to type of therapist. Results indicated that the 959 blacks compared to a 10% random sample of 1190 whites (a) represented a different group of clients in demographic characteristics, (b) were no more likely to receive inferior forms of treatment programs, (c) saw paraprofessionals rather than professional personnel, and (d) failed to return after the initial contact at a high rate (i.e. over 50% terminated at this time). The latter two findings persisted irrespective of other demographic differences between blacks and whites. The results are discussed with reference to the adequacy of mental health care to black Americans. Conclusion of the study observes that mental health centers should examine their policies of staff assignment and pay increased attention to the termination rate of black clients. Evidence was found that discrimination against blacks in the mental health system still exists, albeit, subtle, as reflected in personnel assignment and in the number of contacts.

122. Thomas, C.W. "Final Observations and Summary" Public Health Reports 95 (6) (November/December 1980): 560-61.

Discusses problem areas in black mental health. Lists many proposals to help black mental health. Mental health practitioners need culturally corrective education to better diagnose and treat blacks. Community mental health centers should have a social planning component that conducts research on contemporary issues including spiritually enhancing activities. Pressure should be exerted on training institutions and accrediting houses like the American Psychological Association to see that the training of mental health specialists includes study of the psychology of the black experience.

123. Thornton, C. I. and Carter, J.H. "Improving Mental Health Services to Low Income Blacks." Journal of the National Medical Association 67 (2) (1975): 167-70.

The comprehensive community based health center is discussed from the viewpoint that it is one of the most appropriate methods for delivering mental health services to low-income blacks. The organization of these services at the Lincoln Community Health Center in Durham, NC, is described. The availability of professional services was extended through affiliation with area training programs in psychiatry, social work, and psychology. An awareness of the symptoms and treatment of mental illness was developed through weekly seminars for the entire staff, both professionals and paraprofessionals. It is felt that skilled, indigenous workers (paraprofessionals) can evaluate and interpret abnormal behavior within their culture and can assist immensely with diagnosis and management. Two cases are examined which indicate the importance of mental health care as an integral part of any health care system. It is concluded that future mental health centers concerned with blacks should be planned with the assistance of someone familiar with black behavior.

124. Tomelleri, C.J. et.al. "Who are the 'Committed'?" Journal of Nervous and Mental Diseases 165 (4) (October 1977): 288-93.

A record review of patients who were committed by the court during the course of a hospitalization at an acute urban facility was carried out. Court-committed patients represented 4% of total patients admitted during a 2-year period. Black patients and patients over the age of 70 were more likley to reach the stage of a court hearing and be committed. Schizophrenia was the most frequent diagnosis, being present in well over one half of court-committed patients. Approximately one-third of the patients had a hospital stay exceeding 3 months, and transfer to a long term inpatient program occurred significantly more often among court-committed patients as compared to the rest of the hospitalized population. The majority of court-committed patients were eventually returned to the community. About one fifth were placed in intermediate facilities such as boarding or nursing homes. When legal status of previous and subsequent hospitalization of this sample of court-committed patients was examined, a clear predominance of uncomplicated voluntary hospitalization became apparent.

125. Vail, A. "Factors Influencing Lower-Class Black Patients Remaining in Treatment." Journal of Consulting and Clinical Psychology 46 (2) (April 1978): 341.

Early termination from individual therapy in a community mental health clinic was studied with lower-class black patients assigned to therapists who were black or white. The only significant correlate was the interaction between sex of the therapist and sex of the patient. Patients remained longer with a therapist of the opposite sex. No significant correlations were found between remaining in treatment and black patient's attitudes toward whites, patient's perception of therapists' understanding and acceptance or patient-therapist discrepancies in their perception of therapy.

126. Vernon, S.W., Roberts, R.E. and Lee, E.S. "Response

Tendencies, Ethnicity and Depression Scores." American Journal of Epidemiology 116 (3) September 1982): 482-95.

The Center for Epidemiologic Studies Depression Scale was given to a sample of whites, blacks, and Mexican-Americans residing in Alameda County, California in 1978. Scores on the scale were analyzed to see whether a potentially important source of bias called response tendencies affected prevalence estimates and associations between symptom scores and demographic variables. Response tendencies were found to be differentially correlated with symptom scores by ethnic status. However, the effects were not of sufficient magnitude to alter most associations observed between symptom scores and demographic variables. The need for further methodological studies to clarify the definitions of concepts such as "depression" is discussed.

127. Vernon, S.W. and Roberts, R.E. "Prevalence of Treated and Untreated Psychiatric Disorders in Three Ethnic Groups." Social Science and Medicine 16 (17) (1982): 1575-82.

The pattern and overlap of treated and untreated rates of psychiatric symptoms and disorders were examined in a sample of whites, blacks, and Mexican-Americans. In addition, the study compared treatment sources for family or personal problems for the three groups. The results suggest caution in substituting treated for untreated rates and also in interchanging rates based on symptom scales with rates from clinical diagnostic instruments. Underutilization was assessed by linking psychiatric status with reports of help-seeking behavior. Comparisons indicated that all groups underuse services relative to need, but underutilization is greater for blacks and Mexican-Americans. With the exception of nonpsychiatric physicians, use of treatment sources was similar for all groups. Whites were much more likely than blacks or Mexican-Americans to use this source of care. Possible reasons for this difference are discussed in the context of the methodology employed in the study.

128. Walters, G.D., Greene, R.L. and Jeffery, T.B. "Discriminating Between Alcoholic and Nonalcoholic Blacks and Whites on the MMPI." Journal of Personnel Assessment 48 (5) (October 1984): 486-88.

Investigates the influence of race (black, white) on the MMPI performance of alcoholic and nonalcoholic inpatients. Subjects were 73 (27 black, 46 white) male alcoholic inpatients and 73 (27 black, and 46 white) male nonalcoholic psychiatric inpatients. While black and white alcoholics failed to differ on the MMPI, white alcoholics presented as less disturbed and black alcoholics as less defensive and distressed, compared to their respective nonalcoholic counterparts. Furthermore, only white alcoholics were accurately identified by the MMPI 2-4/4-2 high-point pair combination and only white alcoholics achieved more high-point pairs containing Scale 4 relative to nonalcoholic controls.

129. Watkins, B.A., Cowan, M.A. and Davis, W.E. "Differential Diagnosis Imbalance as a Race-Related Phenonmenon." Journal of Consulting and Clinical Psychology 31 (2) (April 1975): 267-68.

Examines the effect of race, both independent of and interacting with education as a determinant of psychiatric diagnosis. Differential diagnoses were examined in equal numbers of black and white first and second admissions to a psychiatric facility. Black patients were found to have received a significantly higher proportion of schizophrenic diagnoses. This difference remained at all educational levels which suggests that in some cases diagnosis is a function of racial group rather than purely of social class and its attendant factors.

130. White, M.G. The Quality of the Residential Environment as a Social Problem: Empirical Findings on the Mental Health Consequences of Poor Housing and Neighborhood. (Society for the Study of Social Problems, 1983).

Criteria for evaluating the quality of residential environment were developed by the American Public Health Association in the 1940s and became the benchmark by which "slums" and "deteriorating" neighborhoods were defined. At the time, their consequence for the health well-being of residents was assumed. Over the past twenty-five years, researchers have attempted to test this assumption empirically. Results from a recent study of the mental health consequences of poor housing neighborhood are presented. Data were gathered from a 5-year panel study of 350 black and Hispanic low-income females living in Waterbury, Conn. The effects of both general housing and neighborhood conditions as well as specific conditions (crowding, pests, crime) were tested. While neighborhood quality was a more significant factor in poor mental health than housing quality, in general the findings were in line with previous research. Questions about the future of research in this area are raised and some possible changes and their implications are examined.

131. Williams, S.J. et.al. "Mental Health Services: Utilization by Low Income Enrollees in a Prepaid Group Practice Plan and in an Independent Practice Plan." Medical Care 17 (2) (February 1979): 139-51.

Mental health services were included in a comprehensive package of benefits available to low income enrollees in a prepaid group practice plan (PGP) and in an independent practice plan (IPP) under the Seattle

Prepaid Health Care Project There were no out-of-pocket costs for enrollees. Utilization of services was studied for four years under conditions that might stimulate universal entitlement. The analyses indicated that females used substantially more mental health services than males and that enrollees aged 20-44 used more services than those in other age groups. The prepaid group practice generally experienced higher utilization than the prepaid independent plan. Significant racial differences were evident with whites using more services than blacks and black males using strikingly few services. The prepaid independent plan was oriented toward physician providers and emphasized individual psychotherapy while the prepaid group practice employed a diversity of practitioners and therapeutic modalities. The data indicated that the percentage of enrollees using any mental health services was twice as great in the PGP as in the IIP. However, once access to the provider system was achieve, the number of services utilized was greater in the PGP. Inpatient services were also examined. A significantly higher proportion of IPP enrollees were admitted for inpatient care as compared to PGP enrolls. Finally, the cost of mental health services was less than ten percentage of total health service costs in both plans.

132. Wolf, A.M. "A Personal View of Black Inner-City Foster Families." American Journal of Orthopsychiatry 53 (1) (January 1983): 144-51.

The impact of the family unit and family ties among blacks cannot be underestimated when determining health and social needs of individuals. This study uses the observations of a 21 year old white, middle-class, medical student living within a black, inner-city neighborhood to explore the implications of the "extended family" control over individuals. Mental health care and provision of services by mental health providers should respect the special strengths of family ties, particularly in an extended-family situation, if they are to act in the best interests of the children and family members they serve. The observational study focuses upon foster-parent families within Philadelphia's inner-city communities.

133. Wood, W.D. et.al, "Request for Outpatient Mental Health Services: A Comparison of Whites and Blacks." Comparative Psychiatry 25 (3) (May-June 1984): 329-34.

Provides historical information involving blacks and mental health care. The study was conducted through questionnaires given to 309 registrants in adult outpatient service of a university affiliated psychiatric institute. Provides descriptive information of group studied. Study was to provide data on whether white and black requests for mental health services differ. Results indicates whites and blacks differed significantly on four types of requests each rated as more important among blacks. Discussion indicates race is an independent factor and is important in understanding different emphasis placed by blacks and whites in a variety of potential service requests.

134. Yamamoto, J. and Steinberg, A. "Ethnic, Racial, and Social Class Factors in Mental Health." Journal of the National Medical Association (3) (March 1981): 231-40.

A review of the literature reveals that minorities have generally tended to be excluded from the scholarly evaluation of social class factors in alcoholism, drug abuse, and mental illness. When minorities were considered, they were too often misunderstood in terms of negative stereotypes that not only prevail in society, but also influence professionals. When scholarly studies have been done to determine what happens to minority patients in treatment, the findings usually indicate unequal treatment which has not considered the specific subcultural backgrounds and needs of this group. Emphasizes the need for better studies of epidemiology, diagnosis, prevention, treatment, and utilization relating to the minorities and lower class.

3. Health Care Problems

135. Andreopoulos, S. Primary Care: Where Medicine Fails (New York: John Wiley and Sons, 1974).

   A major focus of the book is disparities in health care between the races and reasons why the disparities exist. The author cites an example using the phrase "Ten dollars sick." In Watts, Los Angeles a person has to be sick enough to pay the ten dollar taxi fare or face several hours of bus travel to the county hospital. The point is as distance increases service use tends to decrease. Also identifies difference in Medicare benefits by race. Whites tend to fare better on Medicare reimbursement than blacks. Notes that black elderly persons make the greatest use of hospital outpatient services and that they tend to be poorer than their white counterparts.

136. Argeriou, M. and Zinkowski, J. "Black Alcoholism: A Comment on NIAA's Plan to Combat the Problem." Journal of Studies on Alcohol 37 (7) (July 1976): 1003-09.

   The National Institute on Alcohol Abuse and Alcoholism's Interim Guidelines for the Establishment of Black Alcoholism Projects are criticized for their possible latent function of redirecting treatment energies away from the primary problem of alcoholism.

137. Barber, J.B. "Health Status of the Black Community," Journal of the National Medical Association 71 (1) (January 1979): 87-90.

   Discusses the primary concern of the health status of the black community and provides data on nine points to verify the need for a primary concern among black citizens based on data available. Compares the impact of these conditions on the black community as compared to the white community. Identifies the factors which cause the health care inaccessibility, inadequate prevention of illness, inadequate delivery of health care to poor. Illustrates past achievements undertaken to improve the status of black health care by National Medical Association and endorsement of seventeen proposals for private agencies and government to improve the status of black health care.

138. Brandt, E.N. "Infant Mortality--A Progress Report" <u>Public Health Reports</u> 99 (3) (May/June 1984): 284-88.

Reviews infant mortality rate (I.M.R.) data as of 1981. Points out reasons for higher I.M.R. in the black community. Notes overall decline of I.M.R. in the black community. The provisional infant mortality rate for 1983 is 10.9 deaths per 1000 live births, the lowest rate in history. The U.S. infant mortality rate has been declining at a rapid pace since the late 1960's. In 1981, the latest year in which race-specific data are available, the national I.M.R. was 11.9 per 1000 live births, but the I.M.R. was 10.5 for white infants and 20.0 for black infants. These rates represent I.M.R. declines from 1980 of 4.5 percent for whites and 6.8 percent for black infants. The author states that black mothers are twice as likely as white mothers to deliver a low birth weight infant. Several reasons are: high proportions of teenage pregnancy and out-of-wedlock births; low socioeconomic status; high incidence of anemia and hypertension; and lack of adequate nutrition. The author cites several important principles which have possibly led to a steady narrowing of black-white gap since 1970. Assuming the same average percent decline for I.M.R. of the past decade continues, the projected estimate of I.M.R. for the nation as a whole will fall well within the 1990 target of nine infant deaths per 1000 live births. This yields a rate for black infants of 13.5 as opposed to the target of 12 deaths per 1000 live births.

139. Brink, S.G. and Nader, P.R. "Patterns of Primary Care Utilization in a Triethnic Urban Population of School Children." <u>Medical Care</u> 19 (6) (June 1981): 591-99.

Patterns of primary health care utilization for a random sample of urban elementary school children in three ethnic groups are described. Visit type, reasons for visit, and frequency of visits remained stable from year to year. More than 50 percent of these children were non-visitors each year; 72 percent of those not visiting the first year also did not visit the second year.
Anglo-Americans were more likely to be non-visitors. Enrollment in a children and youth project is examined as a system factor that enabled limited-income families to seek comprehensive medical services. Analysis of the lowest two social classes indicated that significantly fewer Anglos than Mexican-Americans and blacks were enrolled in the Children and

Youth Project. The proportion of Anglo non-visitors in the enrolled group was higher than the proportion of enrolled non-visitors in the Mexican-American and black population. Each year, significantly more children in the non-visitor category were in the non-enrolled group regardless of ethnicity.

140. Cavenar, J.O., Jr. and Spaulding, J.G. "When the Psychotherapist is Black." American Journal of Psychiatry 135 (9) (September 1978): 1084-87.

The authors present a case report of a white neurotic man treated in long-term psychoanalytic therapy by a black woman psychiatrist. The defense mechanism of reversal--the therapist was white in the patient's early dreams--was evident not only in this but in several other white patients treated by the black therapist. The authors suggest that, contrary to the opinions of a few other authors, the reality issues of racial differences can be dealt with successfully in this kind of interracial psychotherapy.

141. Carter, J.H. "Treating Black Patients: The Risk of Ignoring Critical Social Issues." Hospital and Community Psychiatry 32 (4) (April 1981): 281-82.

Examines the development of CMHC facilities in the U.S. Identifies the negative feeling among politicians, public and elite of psychiatric profession. Argues that expansion of services was without special provisions for racial and ethnic minorities. An assumption was made that expansion would meet the needs of minorities. Major failure in providing adequate black health care is due to the "failure to recognize the need for diversity of expertise." Preventive medicine is identified as needing more attention in the U.S. Change from training orientation towards disease needs to be replaced by health oriented training for physicians. Offers recommendations for steps to be followed in the 1980's to serve blacks appropriately.

142. Centennial Program Committee and Department of Preventive Medicine and Public Health, College of Medicine, Howard University, Centennial Conference on the Health Status of the Negro Today and in the Future (Washington, D.C., Howard University Press, 1967).

This report provides information on the analysis of black health, what state it was in in 1967, what were the factors leading to this state, the reasons for the existence of the conditions which existed and recommendations for establishing a means to improve the health conditions and use of health care through education of the recipients, and a need for both the public and private sector to be involved in improving the conditions and and standards of health as they existed in 1967.

144. Clifford, P. and Rene', A. "Substance Abuse Among Blacks: An Epidemiological Perspective" Urban League Review 9 (2) (Winter 1985/86): 52-58.

The actual prevalence of different forms of substance abuse has probably been underestimated in the black community. Problematic drug abuse has been frequently correlated with race/ethnicity. The negative impact of social inequities is reflected in overall poorer health status of black Americans. Medical and social epidemiological data show that increased risk of premature mortality and morbidity are associated with substance abuse.

145. Coney, J.C. The Precipitating Factors in the Use of Alcoholic Treatment Services: A Comparative Study of Black and White Alcoholics (San Francisco: R and E Research Associates, Inc., 1977).

Examines the circumstances under which black and white alcoholics utilize the same treatment program. Develops social and demographic profiles of the participants. Argues that the profiles would serve as background comparisons of the two groups in terms of specific conceptual contructs of alcoholic treatment precipitants. The disparity of usage between blacks and whites of alcoholic treatment programs created the concern for the author to explore th issue. The interplay of social classes regarding prevalence of usage of treatment centers is also examined. It was found that organic therapy and custodial care without treatment were most prevalent in thelower classes while psychotherapy was predominate in the upper classes. Additionally, found that although race was not significantly related to the amount of legal involvement among the study group, more blacks than whites were initiated into treatment through the courts.

146. Cooper, R. et.al. "Improved Mortality Among U.S. Blacks, 1968-1978: The Role of Antiracist Struggle." International Journal of Health Services 11 (4) (1981): 511-22.

A marked improvement in health status for black adults took place over the last decade in the United States. Life expectancy for black men increased 4.6 years between 1968 and 1978, while for black women the increase was 5.7 years. Death rates for the age group 35-74 decreased approximately 25 percent for blacks over the same period. The largest contribution to this improvement was made by cardiovascular diseases (coronary heart disease and stroke). Although similar improvement was observed in the white population, on both a percentage and absolute basis, the change was greater for blacks. For the first time in the U.S., important progress was made in the effort to narrow the gap in mortality rates between black and white adults. Hypertension detection and control appears to have played the key role in this positive public health trend. The community-based demand for greater access to medical care, which emerged from the social struggle of the 1960s also can be accorded a major social role. The current policies of the Reagan Administration pose a serious threat to these antiracist programs, as well as to the effort to close the gap in black-white mortality.

147. Cornely, P. B. "The Health Status of the Negro Today and in the Future." American Journal of Public Health 58 April 1968): 647-54.

Major health problems of black Americans are reviewed. Discussion focuses on the urgency of the black health care situation, the nature of black health problems and some possible solutions to the problems.

148. Eng, E., Hatch, J. and Callan, A. "Institutionalizing Social Support Through the Church and into the Community." Health Education Quarterly 12 (1) (Spring 1985): 81-92.

The positive influence of social support on such health related outcomes as patient adherence to medical regimens and stress reduction at the worksite has captured the attention of public health reseachers and practitioners alike. Yet, the broader social outcome of building community competence to undertake and sustain health related solutions without constant intervention from professionals still remains elusive. The difficulty may lie with the need to uncover on each occasion the various roles and functions of social support structures that may or may not exist in a given community. The intent would then be to graph an intervention onto these existing roles and functions in order to mirror the naturally occurring social support structures. A conceptual framework that has been used to institutionalize health related activities through the role and function of the black church, as a social unit of identity and solution for rural black communities in North Carolina, is put forth for consideration.

149. Fabrega, H. Jr. and Roberts, R. E. "Ethnic Differences in the Outpatient Use of a Public-Charity Hospital." American Journal of Public Health 62 (July 1972): 936-41.

Elucidates the patterns of use by three ethnic groups in a Southwest public charity hospital. (Anglos, Chicanos, and blacks). Discusses the findings in terms of socioenvironmental factors, the medical care system and ethnic status.

150. Felaer, E. et.al., "The Status of Minority Nurses in Wisconsin." Nursing Research 29 (1) (1980): 60-61.

Discusses the status of minority nurses in Wisconsin. Links the problem of adequate health care for minorities to the specific health problems related to ethnicity or lifestyle. Inadequate improvement is a direct result of the lack of ethnic minority health care providers including nurses. Primary reasons for this were determined to be related to level of education of minority nurses, few role models for young, and the lack of knowledge of non-minority nurses leading to a low level of understanding of the needs of the minority patients.

151. Friedman, E. "Private Black Hospitals: A Long Tradition Faces Change." Hospitals 55(13)(1981): 65-68.

Private hospitals owned and governed by black community interests provided a significant amount of health care to black Americans from the Civil War through the 1960s. Many of them are now closed. Suggests that by the end of the century, there will still be black governed and managed institutions, but they will be dependent on their ability to compete and they will be integrated in terms of staff and patients.

152. Gayles, J.N., Jr. "Health Brutality and the Black Life Cycle." The Black Scholar 5 (May 1972): 2-9.

Addresses the history of health brutalization of black people in the U.S. The painful truth we must face is that blacks are ignored, mistreated, abused, and brutalized by the current health care delivery system in the United States. Health care for blacks has mildly improved compared to the conditions blacks faced as slaves, in which thirty to fifty percent died upon slave ships. Blacks suffer from poorer health, higher mortality rates, higher incidences of major diseases, and lower availability and utilization of medical services than most Americans. If black babies and black mothers are not killed by brutal health conditions prior to or during birth, their lives are shortened with continuous and seriously limiting health problems. Malnutrition has the most damaging effects on a black child, whereas hypertension is the major killer among older blacks. The discussion resorts to percentages and statistics concerning the health care brutalization of blacks.

153. Goldenberg, R.L. "Neonatal Deaths in Alabama, 1970-1980: An Analysis of Birth Weight-- and Race-Specific Neonatal Mortality Rates." American Journal of Obstetrics and Gynecology 145 (5) (1983): 545-52.

Alabama birth and death certificate tapes for the years 1970-1980 were linked and analyzed to determine race-specific birth weight and neonatal mortality rate distributions. The analysis indicated that there were no substantial changes in birth weight distributions which could account for the nearly 50% reduction in the neonatal mortality rate in Alabama during this period. Improvements in the quality of medical care and better access to medical care through re-gionalization of perinatal services are suggested as the major reasons for this improvement.

154. Gordon, M. and Hartin, G. A Survey of Health and the Health Care Utilization Patterns of a Small Rural Black Community (Contract under Department of Health, Education and Welfare, Texas Regional Medical Program, Incorporated, 1975).

Collected data from the local community and compared it with similar national data. The predominately black town of Kendleton, Texas has no medical care facilities so residents must use those of nearby cities. Approximately 27 dentists, 5 medical clinics, and 2 hospitals (but no county hospitals) were available with the area. One area hospital willing to release information was utilized by 37 percent of the Kendleton's residents. Findings of the project show that most of the participants frequented physicians adequately but that oral hygiene or preventive dental practices were poor. Respondents were also questioned as to their hospitalizations or visits to a doctor in the last year, the types of prepaid medical coverage, and barriers such as transportation to obtain medical service. Copies of the survey instruments were included in the report.

155. Griffith, E. H. and Mathewson, M. A. "Communitas and Charisma in a Black Church Service." Journal of the National Medical Association 73(11) (November 1981): 1023-27.

Describes the midweek evening service of an independent black church which employs prayer, testimony, and spirit possession. Compares this religious group experience to the theoretical model of the healing community and emphasizes the concepts of "communitas" and "healing charisma." Suggests that the model of a healing community, as represented by this form of the black church service, represents culturally relevant and functionally therapeutic assets for some black people. It is pointed out that knowledge and understanding of the black church in America has directly suffered from the paucity of attention to this area of study.

156. Hadley, J. and Osei, A. "Does Income Affect Mortality: An Analysis of the Effects of Different Types of Income on Age/Sex/Race Specific Mortality Rates in the United States." Medical Care 20 (9) (September 1982): 901-14.

> Explores whether higher incomes are associated with lower mortality rates and discusses prior research in two ways. First, the issue is analyzed separately for eight adults and four infants, age/sex/race are specific population cohorts. Second, total family income is broken down into several components to discover whether different types of incomes have differential effects on mortality rates. Also explores the problem of the joint effects of education and income on mortality. Conclusion tends to support the hypothesis that higher income is associated with lower mortality rates.

157. Hammonds, Karl E. "Blacks and the Urban Health Crisis." Journal of the National Medical Association 66 (3) (1974): 226-31.

> It is proposed that urban health crisis in American cities is caused by a denial of access to the benefits of medical science because of socioeconomic and cultural forces in the ghettos. The indices which give proof of the urban health crisis lie in the areas of health status, care resources, organizations of services, financing, and planning. It is concluded that the present health care system in America exists to serve its own ends, and that the poor, particularly the Black poor, pay to support the medical empire in America. The vital importance of the urban health crisis challenges present and proposed methods of comprehensive health care delivery.

158. Haughton, J.G. "Municipal Hospitals: Their Relevance to the Black Community." Urban League Review 4 (1) (Summer 1977): 25-28.

> Argues that municipal hospitals in the U.S. are critical to the survival of black people. Municipal hospitals serve as substitutes for doctors particularly in communities that have large black populations. Private hospitals with other interests than those of providing health care to the poor and to those unable to pay if allowed to expand at the expense of municipal hospitals, will not adequately serve the poor and minorities. States and local governments must continue to support municipal hospitals.

159. Holliday, B.G. "Advocacy for Life: Mandates Models and Priorities for Prevention." Public Health Reports 95 (6) (November/December 1980): 558.

> Asserts that black homicide should be given a priority in expending Alcohol, Drug Abuse, and Mental Health Administration prevention funds. Black homicide is embedded in the day-to-day

reality of the black community. The Alcohol, Drug Abuse, and Mental Health Administration has a legislative mandate to support research, demonstration projects, and dissemination efforts related to alcohol and drug abuse. Alcohol and drugs figure in the majority of black homicides. Homicides have emotionally stressful antecedents and consequences, and homicide is the ultimate antithesis of health promotion and human resource development.

160. Howze, D.C. "The Black Infant Mortality Rate: An Unequal Chance for Life" Urban League Review 9 (2) (Winter 1985/86): 20-25.

Argues that low birthweight is a major factor in high infant mortality among blacks. The achievement of an adequate income for all should be the ultimate critical intervention for reducing the low birthweight. Proposing other measures without considering this goal is not likely to alter appreciably the problem of black infant mortality and low birthweight.

161. Jackson, J.J. "Special Health Problems of Aged Blacks." Aging (September/October 1978): 15-20.

Discusses health perceptions, age changes, prevalent diseases, functional health, and the use of health resources as they relate to aged blacks. Argues that perhaps the most significant issue is the conditions under which health resources should be color-blind or color-specific for aged blacks. Health is viewed as a crucial problem for most aged blacks. Concludes that the few Federal attempts to set forth research needs for aged blacks in the past have generally ignored critical participants, including biomedical researchers, epidemiologists, health planners, and health providers experienced in treating aged blacks.

162. Johnson, E.F. "Look At It This Way: Some Aspects of the Drug Mix-Up Problem Among Blacks, Poor, Aged, and Female Patients." Journal of the National Medical Association 70 (11) (October 1978): 745-47.

Observes that elderly blacks have insufficient funds to seek proper medical advice. They frequently diagnose their own physical problems and decide that they are minor ones. They are vulnerable to advertising that purports that a pill or a drug which can be purchased without a doctor's prescription will give relief in a short time. This is especially true of drugs advertised to give relief to arthritis. The inability to read labels with understanding continues to be a problem for blacks with limited education, especially the elderly.

163. Jones, J.H. <u>Bad Blood:
The Tuskegee Syphillis
Experiment</u> (N.Y.: The Free
Press, 1981).

>An account of the U.S.
Public Health Service and
other organizations
involvement in a study of
the effects of untreated
syphilis on 399 black men
in Macon County, Alabama,
in and around the county
seat of Tuskegee. The
study began in 1932 and
continued for forty years.

164. Kane, R., Kasteler, J.M.
and Gray, R.M. <u>The Health Gap:
Medical Services and the Poor</u>
(New York: Springer Publishing
Company, Inc., 1976).

>Correlates health care and
socio-economic status,
education, and poverty
levels. Argues that the
poor treat health care in
a consistent manner to
what the poor feel their
style of life to be,
rarely receiving medical
or dental treatment. As a
result, the poor have
greater and more chronic
incidences of medical
problems than do the
affluent. Notes that
efforts are being made to
promote better health
among the poor by
diminishing social class
differences by increasing
health delivery programs
such as OEO and HEW
Neighborhood Health
Centers, Medicare, Medicaid
Model Cities, and Regional
Medical Programs.

165. Lash, M.E., "Community
Health Nursing in a Minority
Setting." <u>Nurse Clinician of
North America</u> 15 (2) (January
1980): 339-48.

>Examines community health
nursing in a minority
environment. Presents a
conceptual model oulining
the sociocultural factors
that may create an impasse
to effective cross-cultural
counseling which is an
important part of health
nursing. Provides the
generic characteristics of
counseling and discusses
language, class, cultural
areas of concern.
Overall, offers a
framework for
understanding the
different ideologies of
racial and ethnic
minorities and how they
may be understood.

166. Levin, J.S. "The Role of
the Black Church in Community
Medicine." <u>Journal of the
National Medical Association</u> 76
(5) (May 1984): 477-83.

>Historically, the black
church has been the
preserver and the
perpetuator of the black
ethos, the center from
which its defining values
and norms have been
generated, and the autono-
mous social institution
that has provided order
and meaning to the black
experience in the U.S.
The traditional ethic of
community-oriented service
in the black ethos is
highly compatible with the
communitarian ethic of
community medicine. Given
this congruence and the
much-documented fact that
black Americans are an
at-risk and underserved
group regarding health
status indicators and the
provision of preventive
health care, respectively,
the black church is an
extremely relevant locus

for the practice of community medicine.

167. Levy, D.R. "White Doctors and Black Patients: Influence of Race on the Doctor-Patient Relationship." Pediatrics 75 (4) (April 1985): 639-43.

    Effective communication between doctor and patient, a skill not emphasized in medical education programs, is essential for patient satisfaction and optimal patient care. In many teaching hospitals, the doctor is commonly white and middle class and the patient black and indigent. Racial differences, even in the absence of social class differences, may have a negative impact on the quality of the doctor-patient relationship. The impact of racism is reviewed, and recommendations to enhance the relationship between white doctors and black patients are made.

168. Lightfoot, O.B. "Preventive Issues and the Black Elderly: A Bio-Psychosocial Perspective." Journal of the National Medical Association 75 (10) (October 1983): 957-63.

    Case report of the black elderly in the United States. Reveals special needs for this disadvantaged group, particularly psychological and social support programs through public health care modes. Discusses preventive health care projects and program objectives.

169. Markides, K.S. "Mortality Among Minority Populations: A Report of Recent Patterns and Trends." Public Health Reports 98 (3) (May/June 1983): 284-91.

    Reviews the mortality experiences of blacks, Native Americans and Hispanics versus Anglo experience and progress made by Hispanics and Native Americans especially in reduction of infant mortality. Provides discussion relative to the degree of improvement of blacks compared to Anglos and Native Americans, reasons for trends and differences among groups in mortality rates and life expectancy and patterns of mortality by cause.

170. Martin, B.J.W. "Ethnicity and Health Care: Afro-Americans" Ethnicity and Health Care (New York: National League for Nursing 1976): 47-55.

    Discusses specific aspects of health care and blacks and is directed towards health workers who provide services to blacks and to other persons who are interested in interacting with blacks with mutual understanding, compassion, and dignity. Notes health problems associated with blacks include lower life expectancy, high infant mortality, childbirth deaths of mothers, tuberculosis rates, childhood illness death rates, invasive cancer and cancer in situ in women, and hypertension. Observes that blacks possess certain habits and beliefs about nutrition and food consumption stemming from cultural roots during slavery periods. Shopping for food, preparation of foods, and reaction to diet changes are strongly influenced by cultural beliefs. Increased awareness and education among health care providers, making them aware and sensitive to black client needs, beliefs and motivations is necessary.

171. Maypole, D.E. and Anderson R., "Minority Alcoholism Programs: Issues in Service Delivery Models." *International Journal of Addiction* 18 (7) (October 1983): 987-1001.

> Describes how one metropolitan community attempted to set up a program to treat black alcoholics. The effort is analyzed from direct service and administration perspectives. When this program failed, an alternative model was developed. The two programs are compared, and an integrated model for minority community alcoholism services is proposed.

172 "Medical History: The New Provident Medical Center." *Journal of the National Medical Association* 75 (7) (July 1983): 727.

> Discusses the opening of an eight-story addition to the 91-year-old Provident Medical Center in Chicago; the oldest independent black hospital in the United States. The hospital holds several other firsts. It was the first black hospital to receive approval by the American College of Surgeons for full residency training in surgery and the first to establish a nursing school for black students.

173. Milner, M. *Unequal Care: A Case Study of Interorganizational Relations in Health Care* (New York: Columbia University Press, 1980).

> Provides a perspective on the dynamics of the pattern of inequality in the nature of interorganizational relationships between urban health care institutions. Observes that low status institutions exist to take on the unwanted functions and patients that the high status institutions refuse. Examines one side of town of a large city and the differences in medical care offered for people who live in a black ghetto right next to a middle class neighborhood. Three hospitals and their health care are explored: a small, very old and very poor, voluntary hospital in the ghetto; a large, high-quality hospital located in the middle class neighborhood near a large university; and another small hospital which also lacks the quality care of the larger hospital located just inside the ghetto.

174. Nace, E.P., Epidemiology of Alcoholism and Prospects for Treatment." *Annual Review of Medicine* 35 (1984): 293-309.

> This chapter reviews current American drinking

patterns and the prevalence of problems resulting from alcohol use. The general population is discussed first. Then a look at five subgroups within the population is presented. These groups are older adults, adolescents, women, blacks, and Hispanics. For the general population as well as each of the five subgroups, the prospects regarding treatment outcome are discussed.

175. Portnoi, V.A. "Delivery of Geriatric Services to Black Senior Citizens." Journal of the National Medical Association 73 (9) (September 1981): 847-51.

Society in this century faces an unprecedented rapid increase in both the absolute number and the relative proportion of senior citizens among the general population. The problems and needs of the elderly require not only a better quality of services than is available at the present time, but also a particular sensitivity to this population's unique and specific needs. Areas of major concern in care for the black elderly and the need to address them in an innovative andcomprehen- sive fashion are discussed

176. Rahbar, F. et. al. "Prenatal Factors Affecting Perinatal Mortality in Blacks." Journal of the National Medical Association 74 (10) (October 1982): 949-52.

A study of 222 black mothers who gave birth to low-birthweight infants in a tertiary care center showed that prenatal care plays a significant role in perinatal outcome. The effect of prenatal care was especially dramatic in the infants weighing less than 1,500 grams. In addition, maternal age is an important factor when less than 17 years. When a teenage pregnancy is associated with a lack of, or irregular, prenatal care, fetal outcome is compromised. Many researchers have indicated that the factors which cause fetal death are the same factors which contribute to neonatal mortality.

177. Reid, J.D. and et.al. "Trends in Black Health." Phylon 38 (2) (June 1977): 105-16.

Blacks are more likely than whites to die from all the major causes of death except suicide. This is simply one aspect of general disadvantages in health which blacks suffer. Many of these disadvantages are avoidable, being due to differential treatment of blacks. One of the best measures of black/white differences in health is sheer survival, measured by life expectancy. In 1900, blacks had substantially lower life expectancies than whites; these lower life ex- pectancies had significant effects on the structure of the black family, making the extended family necessary to ensure that children were cared for. Life expectancy began

HEALTH CARE PROBLEMS

rising only after World War I. Most age-specific death rates have also declined. The main reason for this increase in life expectancy has been the effective control of infectious diseases. At present, the major causes of death among whites (accounting for 70% of deaths) are heart disease, stroke, and cancer; but these account for only 55% of black male 60% of black female deaths. Homicide, however, is much more important among blacks, accounting for 6% of deaths of blacks males; violent death in general is also more important. Black males have higher mortality rates than black females, and the gap has been increasing. Blacks have made considerable gains in health, but there remains considerable room for improvement.

178. Reid, J.D. and Lee, E.S. "Review of the W.E.B. Dubois Conference on Black Health." Phylon 38 (4) (December 1977): 341-51.

According to members of the Dec. 1976 Atlanta University W.E.B. DuBois Conference, the improvement of black health has ceased in the United States because easy improvements have been accomplished and further change would require economic and class structure changes. Prior to the Civil War, slaves had several health advantages over whites. After World War I there was marked improvement in black health and some advance was made during the New Deal era. Black health is negatively influenced by patterns of childbearing and rearing practices and by economic conditions. To improve black health, social, educational, and occupational conditions must improve. Activists and scientists must cooperate as both research and action are needed.

179. Rene', A. and Clifford, P. "Black and White Differentials in Mortality." Urban League Review 9 (2) (Winter 1985/86): 13-19.

Presents an overview of vital statistics data, with particular emphasis on the difference in health status between the black population and the white population with respect to mortality.

180. Rice, M.F. "The Urban Public Hospital: Its Importance to the Black Community." Urban League Review 9 (2) (Winter 1985/86); 64-70.

The sale of public hospitals to the private sector has several negative implications for health care in the black community. The sale of public hospitals and the growth of for-profit chains means higher hospital costs for the black community.

181. Rice, M.F. "Hospital/Health Facilities and the Hill-Burton Obligations: A Secret from the Black Community" Urban League Review 9 (2) (Winter 1985/86): 39-46.

Discusses the uncompensated care and community service obligations of Title XVI of the Public Health Service Act of 1979. Argues that policy analysts have paid little attention to these two obligations in the black community.

182. Riggs, R.S. and Noland, M.P. "Factors Related to the Health Knowledge and Health Behavior of Disadvantaged Black Youth." Journal of School Health 54 (11) (December 1984): 431-34.

> The purpose of this study was to investigate the real relationship between various factors and the health knowledge and health behavior of disadvantaged black youth. Disadvantaged black male and female youths, age 12 to 17, were surveyed regarding their health knowledge, health locus of control, and health practices. Results of the data analyses using an ANOVA revealed significant differences for scores on the health knowledge test due to sex, age, and health locus of control. Females had higher test means than males, older students had higher knowledge scores than did younger students, and internally-oriented students had higher knowledge scores than did externally-oriented students. No significant interaction was found. An ANOVA on behavior scores revealed a sex by locus of control interaction. Male externals had much lower behavior scores than female externals. A significant interaction also was found betweeen age and health locus of control. Older externals had significantly higher behavior scores than younger externals. Implications for health educators and nurse educators are discussed.

183. Robertson, H.R. "Removing Barriers to Health Care: New York City." Nursing Outlook 17 (September 1969): 43-46.

> A public health nurse perspective that explores poverty patients' attitudes and behaviors and offers recommendations for change.

184. Ruiz, D.S. and Hebert, T.A. "The Economics of Health Care for Elderly Blacks." Journal of the National Medical Association 76 (9) (September 1984): 849-53.

> Examines the costs involved with health care delivery to the elderly black population, trends in hospitalization and individualized care, and the quality of health care given to elderly black individuals in comparison with that received by the general population.

185. Seham, M. "Discrimination Against Negroes in Hospitals." New England Journal of Medicine 271 (October 1964): 940-43.

> Argues that discrimination is less publicized in hospitals than in other health care facilities and discrimination is present in all medical settings including hospitals.

186. Shaw, C.T. "A Detailed Examination of Treatment Procedures of Whites and Blacks in Hospitals." Social Science and Medicine 5 (3) (June 1971): 251-56.

A study to determine if whites and blacks receive equal health care in Professional Activity Study (PAS) Hospitals was done. The basic assumption prior to data analysis was that if hospitals give equal care to all patients with similar infirmities, one would expect that approximately equal tests, conferences and evaluations would be made for each patient. This study was based on a sample of 152,625 patients discharged during January through June, 1968, from small, medium and large PAS hospitals in 4 PAS defined regions of the United States. It attempted to investigate possible differences in treatment of whites and blacks in hospitals by using 15 hospitals' procedures (variables) as comparative arguments of treatment. 2-by-2 tables and chi square tests of significance at the .05 level were used for the statistical analysis. Hospitals were compared by the following PAS defined regions: East, Midwest, South and West. This study showed differences in treatment of whites and blacks in hospitals by size and region. The number of times whites appeared to have advantages over blacks is predominant, but there were many examples of the opposite.

187. Schafft, G. "Research Brief: Nursing Homes and the Black Elderly." The Journal of Long-Term Care Administration 7 (Winter 1979): 35-43.

This study was designed on a case study model. This allowed the research team to best define the issues involving access of the black elderly to long-term care and to develop improved standards for admissions procedures and programs within homes. Barriers to the use of nursing homes by blacks include preferences within the black community, inadequate public financing of nursing home care, and historical and current practices within the health services profession. There are two major reasons for black underrepresentation in nursing homes. First, the black population prefers to care for the elderly at home because of the role blacks play in the family and the unattractiveness of a nursing home. Second, nursing home care is not readily available to the black population in metropolitan areas because of racism and the lack of information. Government agencies and private organizations are attempting an inclusive and humane approach to care for the black portion of the population.

188. Schafft, G. and Yokie, A.J. "Health Care for Racial and Ethnic Minorities and Handicapped Persons." The Journal of Long-Term Care Administration 8 (Winter 1980): 37-40.

Argues that in the last ten years, nursing homes have increased their populations. The black elderly are not fully using these long-term health options to the same extent as the white elderly. The study asserts that black and white elderly can comfortably live together in nursing homes. For the elderly, health status seems to take precedence over racial status. The administrators in the nursing home find it crucial to guarantee equal access and equitable care. There are effective ways for administrators to accomplish such a goal. First, nursing home personnel should make contacts in the black community to let it be known beds are available on a non-discriminatory basis. Second, front office and administrative staffs should be integrated. Thirdly, the administrator should set the tone for integration in the facility. Fourthly, the nursing home should reflect the black experience. Finally, the Board of Directors should be integrated.

189. Shader, R.I and Tracy, M. "On Being Black, Old, and Emotionally Troubled: How Little is Known. Psychiatric Opinion 10 (December 1973): 26-32.

Reviews multiple factors in pursuing answers to questions regarding identification and management of elderly blacks. Black elderly patients comprise only 3.7% of our geriatric inpatient experience. Although many explanations have been considered in evaluation of the low number of black geriatric patients, no single explanation appears to account for the small numbers of elderly blacks. It is probable that several causes contribute in varying degree in various communities. Superimposed on a background of early mortality, these factors could begin to explain the relatively low frequency of black geriatric patients seen in urban psychiatric facilities.

190. Sinkford, J.C. and Henry, J.L. "Survival of Black Colleges from a Dental Perspective." Journal of the National Medical Association 73 (6) (June 1981): 511-15.

Argues that to achieve health for all in the U.S. by the year 2000, as proposed by the World Health Organization, dental health needs must be considered a part of total health. The failure to address dental health needs has reached a crisis level, particularly in the black communities throughout the nation. The dental delivery system in the U.S. requires a continuous upgrading of the quality of education for those who will be the deliverers of dental services in the future. In order to accomplish this, we must utilize fully the present academic system to assure access, quality, and availability of dental health care for all Americans in the future.

191. Watts, T.D. and Wright, R. Black Alcoholism: Toward A Comprehensive Understanding (Springfield, IL.: Charles C. Thomas, 1983).

Adopts a preventive perspective, critiques a variety of theories used to explain alcoholism among blacks, and describes briefly the issue of treatment. It is replete with theoretical frameworks and ways to conceptualize alcoholism. But it is relatively short on practical suggestions or insights about ways to handle the problem. This book focuses the attention of researchers and practitioners on this important problem and prepares the way for systematic clinical research.

192. Weaver, J.L. "Personal Health Care: A Major Concern for Minority Aged." Comprehensive Service Delivery System For The Minority Aged. E. Percil Standford (ed). (San Diego, California: Center on Aging, School of Social Work, San Diego State University, 1977): 41-62.

Argues that poverty, discrimination, segregation and little or no access to health care providers seem to have produced a selected body of elderly -- perhaps only the strong survive -- because the mortality picture of very old blacks (Over 75 years) is generally better than that of their Anglo peers. Nevertheless, for all black elderly, there is a persistent pattern of higher incidence of most chronic diseases, days of forced inactivity, and visits to physicians. Studies which combine non-elderly with elderly are misleading, while studies of black elderly alone document conditions without offering a yardstick for determining the relative severity or frequency of problems for blacks. The most severe health problem of the black elderly and for the overall black community is hypertension.

193. Wilson, J.L. "Geriatric Experiences With the Negro Aged." Geriatrics 8 February 1953): 88-92.

While there are no sharp differences in the majority of diseases affecting the black aged and those affecting whites in the same age bracket, there are certain differences in etiologic factors and incidence of ailments which merit consideration and correction. Six of the fourteen diseases encountered, using a Negro population between the ages of 55 and 91, were (1) cardiovascular diseases, with or without hypertension; (2) arteriosclerosis, generalized; (3) hypertrophic and infectious arthritis and osteoarthritis; (4) calcified fibroma uteri; (5) hypertrophied prostate; and (6) carcinoma of breast, uterus and stomach. Factors determining the incidence of certain ailments in aged blacks are primarily economic. Where they exist, a low wage scale and long working hours tend to undermine body resistance. Poor housing, overcrowding, and unsanitary conditions increase infectious diseases. Inadequate diet promotes low serum proteins which retard tissue repair. In certain areas of the country some hospitals refuse to admit blacks, who in many instances are not hospitalized when necessary. Also of significance is the refusal of several medical schools to give postgraduate and refresher courses to black physicians.

194. Wilson, P.A. et.al. "Does Race Affect Hospital Use?" American Journal of Public Health 5 (3) (March 1985): 263-69.

Based on 1980 hospital discharges in areas in the State of Michigan with substantial black populations. Blacks use approximately 50 percent more hospital care than whites, but about half this difference is associated with use in specific communities, which affects both white and black use. Black use is not associated with community size, percentage of blacks, or available beds and doctors. After controlling for mortality and socioeconomic status, a small statistically non-significant difference in race-specific use remains for 23 Michigan communities. The elimination of race as an explainer of hospital use suggests progress in assuring equal access to hospitals, but differences in poverty, mortality, and some specifics of use remain.

195. Wolf, J.H. et.al. "Access of the Black Urban Elderly to Medical Care." Journal of the National Medical Association (January 1983): 41-6.

Provides statistical data on the rates of hypertension, diabetes, and arthritis in blacks 65 years of age and older for 1977. Also provides a demographic and socioeconomic profile of elderly urban blacks, addresses health status of individuals, methods of health care include sources and utilization, and determinants of health care utilization by the surveyed community.

196. Yabura, L. "Health Care Outcomes in the Black Community." Phylon 38 (2) (June 1977): 194-202.

Poverty and ill health are mutually reinforcing phenomena. Hunger and malnutrition, predominantly affecting the poor, produce mental and physical disabilities limiting the chance to escape poverty. Life expectancies are about 10% lower for blacks Hypertension in particular is a very important disease among blacks, more than twice as common as among whites. There is a need for an active integrated, coordinated and comprehensive health policy to deal with this problem. In particula blacks need to be integrated into the health care system. The institution of national health insurance would not significantly change this. What is needed is a national health care system in which control of health care belongs to those who receive it.

62. Yankauer, A. "Black Physicians and Black Communities." <u>American Journal of Public Health</u> 67 (6) (June 1977): 511-12.

An editorial which provides a review of Dr. Lois Gray's article, "The Geographic and Functional Distribution of Black Physicians: Some Research and Policy Considerations." Provides a review of statistical data and information relative to the concentrations of black physicians in urban areas, discusses reasons for selection of areas served by black physicians, discusses future preventive medicine trends for blacks and addresses need for policies which are aimed at the desires and needs of the patients as opposed to correcting the maldistribution of physicians.

4. Assessment Studies

198. Armstrong, H. "Nutritional Status of Black Preschool Children in Mississippi: Assessment by Food Frequency Scale." Journal of the American Dietetic Association 66 (5) (May 1975): 488-93.

Food frequency data were studied in relation to the nutritional status of 372 black preschool children in three Mississippi counties. The following data were utilized: quantitative dietary intakes for four or seven days from which intakes of eight nutrients and energy were calculated; frequency of consumption of all individual foods was obtained; and anthropometric (height) and biochemical (Hemoglobin) measures. Six Guttman scales of food consumption frequencies were constructed. In four scales, all foods consumed in four or seven days were assigned to one of nine food groups which formed scale steps. Kendall's tau correlations coefficents were calculated for relationships between all scales and commonly used indicators of nutritional status, including calculated intakes of eight nutrients and energy, height percentiles, and hemoglobin values. Two total food consumption scales based on seven-day dietary intakes were valid indicators of nutritional status, i.e., the scales were significantly correlated with all three indicators of nutritional status. This research focused on relationship between the food scales and nutritional status indicators as an initial step in a study of overall family development. The food scale alone, which has meaning for both the nutritionist and the sociologist, has implications for nutrition education in determining what to teach, selecting teachers, and evaluating change in food practices.

199. Benjamin, R. and Benjamin, M. "Social Correlates of Black Drinking: Implications for Research and Treatment." Journal of Studies on Alcohol Supplement 9 (January 1981): 241-45.

Black college students in Mississippi were part of a study which concluded that negative parental attitudes toward drinking did not necessarily result in children becoming abstainers. Drinking tended to be done for utilitarian purposes and students had negative attitudes toward drinking. The study argues that research on blacks should take into account their historical and contemporary positions in society. Race is considered an important variable in any study of alcohol use and misuse. A black drinker may become the object of racial hatred and intolerance in addition to any negative judgement toward the drinking behavior. Alcohol abuse is the number one health problem and number one social problem in black America. Race is also a factor in determining the quality of treatment an alcoholic will receive. Blacks were found to be underrepresented in all treatment programs and the quality of treatment received was not comparable to that received by whites. The authors suggest that more attention must be given to the following in order to study blacks and alcohol: 1) Measures of Alcohol Use and Misuse from Black Minority Group Perspectives; 2) The Impact of Alcohol Overuse; 3) The Management of Alcohol Overuse on Family Members and Friends; and 4) Intraracial Comparisons of Perception of Alcohol Misuse.

200. Blake, J.H. "'Doctor Can't D Me No Good." Social Concomitants of Health Care Attitudes and Practices Among Elderly Blacks in Isolated Rural Populations." The Black Sociologist (8) (1-4) (Fall/Summer 1978-79): 6-13.

Observations and interviews with elderly black residents of Sea Islands, Ga show generally negative attitude toward medical practitioners and a disinclination to follow prescribed treatment regimens. Hospitals are strongly associated with death and are used only as a last resort. Physicians are suspected of having little knowledge of nature, with which islanders closely identify and venerate as the true source of life, sustenance, and health. Cultural value placed on knowledge of ocean tides, farming lore, folk remedies, and "participation" in nature's ways should be weighed carefully in medical policies regarding the rural elderly.

201. Boyer, E. "Variations in Health Perceptions Between Black and White Elderly." International Quarterly of Community Health and Education 2 (2) (1981/82): 157-73.

In a sample of 414 residents of public housing for the elderly, black residents (number of cases = 100) evaluated their own health significantly lower than did whites (number of cases = 314). The relationship of perceived health to several measures of objective health status, cultural background, social participation, and morale was analyzed separately for the two ethnic groups. The relationship of measures of health to health perception is more direct among whites than blacks except for an Index of Daily Well-Being in which the relationship is similar for both groups. Social participation was also found to influence health perception. With blacks, participation in church-related activities is the most direct influence. While health perception is related to morale, life orientation (an index of morale) is higher for blacks than for whites. The implications for health education professionals seem to lie in the lack of direct links between objective measures of health and self-perception of health for blacks. The need for health education to facilitate realistic self-appraisal of health conditions is evident. The relatively low educational levels of many older citizens, especially blacks, suggests that news paper announcements are no longer an adequate source of health information for the elderly.

202. Brunswick, A.F. "Health Stability and Change: A Study of Urban Black Youth." American Journal of Public Health 70 (5) (May 1980): 504-13.

Reports on a study conducted with 536 urban black youths at two points in life, at adolescence, ages 12-17, and at adulthood, ages 18-23. Questions related to 47 health problems, the incidence of these problems in both groups and the extent of of change which occurred, the direction of change, and the health problems most subject to change. Offers a comparison of the number of problems which increased for both sexes and a comparison of the increase of problems between male and female participants.

203. Brunswick, A.F. and Messeri, P. "Casual Factors in Onset of Adolescents' Cigarette Smoking: A Prospective Study of Urban Black Youth." Advances in Alcohol and Substance Abuse 3 (1-2) (Fall 1983/Winter 1984): 35-52.

This research is based on a two-wave panel study of 536 urban black adolescents. Six to eight years intervened between measuring the predictors and measurement of subsequent smoking initiation. Separate prediction models were tested for males and females, based on a multivariate causal model which spanned five domains of prior conditions: personal background, school achievement, family-peer orientations, psychogenic orientations, and health attitudes and behaviors. Variables from all five domains influenced subsequent smoking but different predictors were implicated for adolescent males vs. females. This lends support to one of the major hypotheses in this research--that the salient experiences which governed the decision to start smoking were different for black males and females. Applying the same prediction model to cigarette smoking and to illicit drug involvement showed no overlap in prediction for males and all but two of the same influences were significantly implicated in females' illicit drug use and cigarette smoking.

204. Caetano, R. "Ethnicity and Drinking in Northern California: A Comparison Among Whites, Blacks and Hispanics." Alcohol and Alcoholism 19 (1) (1984): 31-44.

This research reports the drinking patterns and alcohol problems in three ethnic groups of the U.S. population: whites, blacks, and Hispanics. Respondents were sampled randomly from the general population of three counties of the San Francisco Bay Area in Northern California. Both black and Hispanic females have higher rates of abstention than white females, but at the aggregate level males drinking patterns are similar across ethnic groups. However, among males the pattern of drinking and the prevalence of alcohol problems by age change dramatically according to ethnicity. Among white males drinking and problems decrease abruptly from the twenties to the thirties, as has been traditionally found in the U.S. general population. Among black males the trend is exactly the opposite of that for whites, while among Hispanic males there also is a decrease, but not quite so large as that for whites, and the frequency of heavy drinking and problems is always higher than for the other two groups. The types of problems reported by respondents do not vary by ethnicity but the sociodemographic correlates of both number of drinks consumed per month and number of alcohol problems do differ among the ethnic groups. Both Hispanics and blacks have more liberal attitudes toward alcohol use than whites. These results suggest that whites, blacks and Hispanics each have a characteristic way of using alcoholic beverages. The less restrictive views toward alcohol use in the black and Hispanic culture, as well as the different patterns of drinking and problems by age, are of importance for prevention. Whites, blacks and Hispanics have different groups of people at risk for developing alcohol problems and prevention should be planned accordingly.

205. Callender, C.O. et.al. "Attitudes Among Blacks Toward Donating Kidneys for Transplantation: A Pilot Project." Journal of the National Medical Association 74 (8) (August 1982): 807-9.

Patients requiring kidney transplants have three possible sources: (1) a kidney from an individual who dies suddenly (approval for the transplant must be given by the next-of-kin of the deceased); (2) a kidney from a relative; and (3) a kidney from one who "willed" it to be transplanted following his or her death. Each of these circumstances requires decision making. On the basis of this information, a research program designed to determine the nature of attitudes of blacks toward kidney donations was developed. Results disclosed a lack of knowledge about kidney transplantation, disassociation and lack of communication between blacks and the medical community; religious fears; fears of premature death; and racism.

206. Cartwright, S. "Report on the Diseases and Physical Pecularities of the Negro Race." New Orleans Medical Journal (May 7, 1851).

Argues that behavioral differences between whites and blacks could be explained on anatomical and physiological grounds. Reports that blacks have a smaller brain than whites and have a peculiar and innate disposition to rhythm as compensation for their lack of intellectual abilities. Notes that blacks are prone to specific diseases, including "negro consumption" and "drapetomania" causing blacks to break, waste and destroy everything they handle.

207. Centerwall, B.S. "Race, Socioeconomic Status, and Domestic Homicide, Atlanta, 1971-72" American Journal of Public Health 74 (8) (August 1984): 813-815.

Analysis of 222 intra-racial domestic homicides (186 blacks and 36 white victims) committed in Atlanta in 1971-72. A domestic homicide is defined as a criminal homicide committed in a residence by a relative or acquaintance of the victim. When black and white populations were compared for rates of household crowding, the relative risk of intra-racial domestic homicide in black populations was no longer significantly elevated. Using rates of household crowding as an index of socioeconomic status, blacks were no more likely to commit domestic homicide than were whites in comparable socioeconomic circumstances.

208. Chee, P. and Kane, R. "Cultural Factors Affecting Nursing Home Care for Minorities: A Study of Black American and Japanese-American Groups." Journal of the American Geriatrics Society 31 (2) (February 1983): 109-12.

In a pilot study of two nursing homes serving primarily different ethnic groups, differences were found in the importance black patients and their relatives attached to the ethnic character of the institution compared with respondents in a Japanese home. The latter placed more emphasis on all aspects of ethnic programming and homogeneity of patients and staff. Blacks placed more emphasis on access to family than on ethnic orientation per se. Concern is expressed about the need for better understanding of how cultural and social factors may play a role in the way different ethnic minority groups care for their elderly.

209. Cooper, R. "A Note on the Biologic Concept of Race and its Application in Epidemiologic Research."

American Heart Journal 108 (3) (Part 2) (September 1984): 715-22.

Use of the category of race in epidemiologic research presupposes scientific validity for a system that divides man into subspecies. Although the significance of race may be clear-cut in many practical situations, an adequate theoretical construct based on biologic principles does not exist. Anthropologists have in large measure abandoned the biologic concept of race, and its persistent widespread use in epidemiology is a scientific anachronism. The assumption that race designates important genetic factors in a population is in most cases false. Racial definitions should be seen as primarily social in origin and should be clues to environmental-rather than genetic-causes of disease. An understanding of the social forces leading to racial differentials in health will give further direction to preventive campaigns.

210. Davidson, D.W. and Spollen, J.J. "The Influence of Clinical Judgement on the Rate of Referrals from School Vision Screening Program", Journal of the American Optometrists Association 50 (10) (October 1979): 1126-27.

Investigates clinical judgement and its influence on the proportion of referrals as a result of ethnicity and socioeconomic income levels. Findings based on observations in Alabama of black preschool children from low income families and their above-average rate of referral from a school vision screening program. Observes that a contributing factor to the high rate of referrals was that examiners may have often modified the referral criteria based on their clinical judgement. Findings, however, indicate modification of referral criteria does not significantly influence the proportion of referrals based on ethnicity and socio-economic income level of families.

211. Decker, D.L. and Caetano, D.F. "Variations in Natal Knowledge Among High School Students." Journal of School Health 47 (5) (May 1977): 286-88.

An itemized questionnaire on natal knowledge was given in a high school sample in which there was a large diverse racial and ethnic population. The results of the study indicated that there are statistical significant differences between racial and sexual groups in the level of natal knowledge. Whites had the largest proportion of high scores followed by blacks and Mexican-Americans. The differences from male to female were more outstanding, with females scoring much higher than males. The data indicate that in the sample of high school students there are significant differences in the level of natal knowledge of different racial and ethnic groups.

212. Driscoll, D.P. and Royster, L.H. "Comparison Between the Median Hearing Threshold Levels for An Unscreened Black Nonindustrial Noise Exposed Population (NINEP) and Four Presbycusis Data Basis." *American Industrial Hygiene Association Journal* 45 (9) (1984): 577-93.

The median hearing threshold level (HTL) data representing an unscreened black nonindustrial noise exposed population (NINEP) are compared to the median HTL data of three previously established presbycusis data bases, which are all normalized relative to age 18. Comparisons are made betweeen the black NINEP and the presbycusis data based HTLs for different sex and age groupings. The unscreened black NINIP exhibits median HTLs similar to those of the presbycusis data bases for ages less than approximately 35-45 years. However, for age groupings greater than 35-45, the median HTLs of the black NINEP are generally lower (better hearing) than those of the referenced presbycusis data bases.

213. Durant, R.H. et.al. "The Relationship Between Physical Activity and Serum Lipids and Lipoproteins in Black Children and Adolescents." *Journal of Adolescent Health Care* (3) (1983): 55-60.

Assesses the association between the serum lipid and lipoprotein levels of 62 black children and 37 black adolescents and their reported levels of habitual physical activity, 24-hour dietary intake and physical measurements. In the children physical activity was not correlated with serum lipid and lipoprotein levels. In the adolescents, high-activity subjects had lower total serum cholesterol/high-density-lipoprotein cholesterol ratios than less active subjects. Results suggest that increased habitual physical activity may have a favorable effect on serum lipid and lipoprotein levels in black adolescents.

214. Edwards, G.F. *The Negro Professional Class* (Westport, CT.: Greenwood Press, 1982): Chapter 5.

The author examines the Negro professional through social trend analyses of current data. Social structure and motivational patterns are explored to learn how professions as physicians, dentists, lawyers, and teachers compared with each other. The favored occupation was that of a medical doctor. Survey respondents favored this occupation for themselves as well as being the desired field for children to enter. Chief influences of those blacks entering the medical profession were family influence, interest in work, and encouragement by someone other than a teacher, in that order. Other contributing motivators included opportunity for service (6.7 percent), financial rewards (5.6 percent), desire for independence (5.6 percent), the prestige of the profession (3.3 percent), "unknown" (3.3 percent), and best opportunity at time of beginning (2.2 percent). Also discusses the chief sources of financial assistance for meeting college and professional expenses, academic rank of physicians in their high school classes, and when the decision was made to enter the medical profession.

215. Edwards, L.N. and Grossman, M. "Income and Race Differences in Children's Health in the Mid-1960's." Medical Care 20 (9) (September 1982): 915-30.

 This article explores income and race differences in eight measures of the health of children ages 6 through 11 as assessed in the early 1960s It is shown that both income and race differences in health are much less pronounced than they are in infant mortality and birth weight data. Significant differences are found in the health status of black and white children and of children from high and low-income families, but these are primarily differences with respect to parent-reported (rather than physician-reported) health criteria and they by no means overwhelmingly favor the white or high-income children. These findings underscore the importance of treating children's health status as multidimensional. In addition, these findings will serve as a bench mark for studies of children's health using data for a more recent period.

216. Egbert, L.D. and Rothman, I. "Relation Between the Races and Economic Status of Patients and Who Performs their Surgery." New England Journal of Medicine 297 (2) (July 14, 1977): 90-91.

 Evaluates the relation between race and economic status of surgical patients and their likelihood of being treated by a surgeon in training as opposed to a staff surgeon. Provides data comparing blacks to whites relative to who provided care, addressed this issue related to the method of payment, and illustrated facts attributing treatment of black emergency patients to surgeons in training.

217. Farmer, M.E. et.al. "Race and Sex Differences in Hip Fracture Incidence." American Journal of Public Health 74 (12) (December 1984): 1374-79.

 Incidence rate for hip fracture in the U.S. are estimated using non-federal hospital discharges from the National Hospital Discharge Survey for the years 1974 to 1979. Age-specific rates by five-year age groups are compared among the four race-sex groups. No significant differences were observed among black males, black females, and white males. In contrast, rates for white females are one and one-half to four times those for black females after age 40 and are double those of white males after age 50. There is no signficant difference between black women and black men. Findings suggest that environmental and/or lifestyle factors, in addition to genetic factors, may play a significant role in determining who sustains a hip fracture.

218. Freeman, E.W. et.al. "Urban Black Adolescents Who Obtain Contraceptive Services Before or After Their First Pregnancy." Journal of Adolescent Health Care 5 (3) (July 1984): 183-90.

Compares three groups of urban black teenagers at their enrollment in a contraceptive program and at a one-year follow-up. The groups comprise 263 never pregnant, postabortion and postpartum teens ages 17 or less at their initial family planning visit. Self-report questionnaires examined attitudes and information about pregnancy and contraceptive use, sources of contraceptive information, sexual and contraceptive experience, family and partner support for contraceptive use, and demographic background factors. These data suggest the need for earlier family involvement in educating and guiding teens together with access to contraceptive services in preventing unwanted adolescent pregnancies.

219. Futrell, M.F., Kilgore, L.T. and Windham, F. "Nutritional Status of Black Preschool Children in Mississippi: Influence of Income, Mother's Education, and Food Programs." Journal of the American Dietary Association 66 (1) (January 1975): 22-27.

The nutritional status of 247 black preschoolers in two counties of Mississippi was studied by relating caloric and nutrient intakes and anthropometric measurements to homemaker's education, family income, and participation in Food Stamp and donated food programs. Low intakes of calories, iron, calcium, vitamin A, and ascorbic acid were found in many of the children, regardless of the variable considered. These findings--in comparison with similar studies--imply that, as time passes, low education and income are having less impact on child nutrition. This ameliorating effect may be due to programs designed to educate parents and extend purchasing power of food dollars. Thus, it seems advisable to continue these programs.

220. Gaines, V.P. "Career Counseling as Experienced." Practicing Black Ophthalmologists." Journal of the National Medical Association 72 (11) (November 1980): 1085-91.

A questionnaire was sent to a random sample of the practicing black ophthalmologists in the country, and the compiled data indicated that the majority of respondents attended all black schools where career counseling per se did not

exist except in the form
of teacher assistance or
parental pressure. At the
college and university
level there was again a
lack of counseling
services and the faculty
served as the motivating
agents.

221. Galloway, N.O. "Medical
Aspects Of the Aging American
Black." Proceedings of Black
Aged In The Future, Jacquelyne
J. Jackson, Editor. (Durham,
N.C.: Center For The Study of
Aging and Human Development,
Duke University, 1973): 50-60.

A brief description of the
overall health of the
black aged and compares
selected non-white with
white life expectancies,
and mortality rates and
causes. Argues that the
black aged represent a
biologically superior
population in comparison
with younger blacks and
aged whites. Concludes
that better health in
younger years will
contribute to longer black
life-expectancies and a
larger population of black
aged.

222. Garn, S.M. and Clark, D.C.
"Problems in the Nutritional
Assessment of Black
Individuals." American Journal
of Public Health 66 (March
1976): 262-267.

Argues that the
nutritional assessment of
black Americans is
complicated by differences
in socioeconomic status.
These include smaller size
at birth but greater size
from 2 to 14 years,
advanced skeletal
development, advanced
dental development, a
larger skeletal mass and
bone density, and a lesser
rate of adult bone loss in
the black female.
Differences in hemoglobin
concentration and in
hematocrit levels also
indicate the need for
population-specific
standards. Since
self-assignments to facial
categories are commonly
used, the problem of racial
identification is minimal.

223. Globetti, G. "Alcohol Use
Among Black Youths in a Rural
Community." Drug and Alcohol
Dependency 2 (4) (July 1977):
255-60.

The results of this study
lead to the conclusion that
the circumstances which
surround the act of youth
drinking in the black
population of an abstinence
setting are somewhat
different from those
recorded elsewhere.
Although fewer students
drink, the drinking styles
reveal several dimensions
frequently associated with
alcohol abuse. As a rule,
users do not have parental
permission to drink and for
the most part they identify
with churches that condemn
alcohol on moral grounds.
Because many of the youth
procure their beverages
from illegal sources or in
an illegal way, they tend
to drink in a surreptitious
manner in a setting absent
of restraint.
Consequently, a significant
number of youths were
drinking without normal
propriety and were
exhibiting several social
complications as a result.
This suggests that less
drinking can be expected in
abstinence settings but

among those young people who drink, problems may be more frequent. This is logical since the user is at variance with the normative prescriptions of the community, church, and home. Obviously, drinking under these conditions may actually be an expression of a general test of the limits of the adult world or a symbol of rejection of adult standards. Subsequently, the abuse of alcohol may decrease with maturity. Regardless of their meaning, however, the findings do point to a need for education about alcohol at the school level.

224. Goldstein, G. et.al. "Withdrawal Seizures in Black and White Alcoholic Patients: Intellectual and Neuropsychological Sequelae." Drug and Alcohol Dependence 12 (1) (1983): 349-63.

An investigation was made to determine whether black alcoholics have a different response to withdrawal seizures than white alcoholics in terms of cognitive and other neuropsychological deficits. The apparently higher incidence of withdrawal seizures among blacks noted during screening of subjects for a previous study raised the question of whether the consequences of the seizure history might be different among blacks. Results of the study indicated that on several tests there were significant differences between black patients with and without seizure histories when compared to whites. Various possible causes for this finding are discussed.

225. Gordon, W.C., Jr. et.al. "A New Look at Peripheral Vascular Disease in Blacks: A Two-Year Update." Journal of the National Medical Association 72 (12) (December 1980): 1177-83.

There is an apparent disproportionate loss of lower extremities to arterosclerotic disease among black patients. A comprehensive overview of 66 patients-the majority of whom were black --undergoing distal lower extremity revascularization for severe arterosclerotic ischemia with impending limb loss is presented. Patients in the study group are presented according to race, sex, and age. Their histories and pre-operative clinical conditions, along with angiographic and operative findings lead to the identification of a previously undescribed arteriosclerotic phenomenon present among blacks. The impact of an aggressive program for limb salvage is reported.

226. Greene, S. and Salber, E. "Racial Differences in Medical Care Expenditures." Medical Care 17 (10) (October 1979): 1029-36.

Examines the out of pocket medical expenditures made by families on a racial basis in a Southern rural community. Findings indicate that white families paid an average of $709.00 per year as compared to $383.00 paid by black families. The differences between black and whites are then viewed with respect to the family's characteristics, race, education of the head of the household, family income, family size and composition. The results of the study show that whites consistently report greater expenditures than blacks. Differences are partly due to a mixture of three factors: 1) variations in the cost of doctor visits to whites; 2) a lower level of use of services by blacks, and 3) the differential availability and use of third party payors.

227. Haigh, N.Z. et.al. "The East Baltimore Study: The Relationship of Lipids and Lipoproteins to Selected Cardiovascular Risk Factors in an Inner City Black Adult Population." American Journal of Clinical Nutrition 38 (August 1983): 320-26.

Low socioeconomic status, inner city black adults, aged 20 to 49 yrs (24 males and 45 females, were randomly selected from East Baltimore, MD to study plasma lipid and lipoprotein levels. Several factors known to affect these levels also were examined: dietary intake, alcohol intake, degree of obesity (measured by body mass index), physical activity level, smoking and hormone use. Compared to women, the men consumed 9.3 more calories/kg body weight ($p<0.005$), 273 mg more cholesterol/day ($p<0.005$), and 7% fewer calories as sucrose ($p<0.01$). The P/S ratio of both their diets was 0.5. The men also had a lower body mass index than the women (23.9 kg/m^2 versus 29.0; $p<0.001$). Mean lipid and lipoprotein levels were similar in the men and women. However, the men's total cholesterol (167 mg/dl) and low density lipoprotein cholesterol 94 mg/dl) levels were lower than those of adult blacks in other studies, while the levels of the East Baltimore women were similar to those in other studies. For women, body mass index and high density lipoprotein cholesterol were negatively correlated ($p<0.01$). None of the factors studied explained the relatively low total cholesterol and low density lipoprotein cholesterol levels in these inner city black adult men.

228. Hawkins, R. "Dental Health of Aged Blacks." Proceedings of Black Aged In the Future. Jacquelyne J. Jackson, Editor. (Durham, N.C.: Center for the Study of Aging and Human Development, Duke University, 1973): 57-77.

There is an alarming number of older blacks needing early dental care. Among those 55-64 years of age, 78.5 percent of black males and 79.2 percent of black females needed such care. Concludes that dental health care is generally poor for most blacks, and it tends to become increasingly poor with age. Points out that those interested in curriculum building for the aged must also be interested in increasing the number of black dentists available to treat aged blacks.

229. Himes, J.H. "Appropriateness of Parent-Specific Stature Adjustment for U.S. Black Children." Journal of the American Medical Association 76 (1) (January 1984): 55-57.

The appropriateness for U.S. black children of a new method that considers parental statures when evaluating a child's length or stature is discussed. Although there are small differences in the average growth of blacks and whites, it is suggested that a single growth standard (the National Center for Health Statistics percentiles) is appropriate for the evaluation of length and stature of black children. Recent national data show no important differences between mean statures of black and white adults that would render the parent-specific method inappropriate for U.S. blacks. The new method is recommended as an aid in determining the nature of statural growth problems.

230. Hochbert, M.C., Linet, M.S., and Sills, E.M. "The Prevalence and Incidence of Juvenile Rheumatoid Arthritis in an Urban Black Population." American Journal of Public Health 73 (October 1983): 1202-3.

Determines the prevalence and incidence of juvenile rheumatoid arthritis (JRA) in an urban black population, identifying three cases through review of computerized outpatient encounters and a fourth case by reviewing discharge records at hospitals. The prevalence of JRA among blacks was estimated as 0.26 per 1,000. The average annual incidence of JRA was 6.6 per 100,000 per year. This data suggests that the black race is not associated with the increased risk of the development of JRA. However, the black race is associated with an increased incidence of and mortality from systemic lupus erythematosus, but not adult onset rheumatoid arthritis.

231. Holmes, D. and Terisi, J.A. Information About, and Attitudes Toward, the Use of Long-term Care and Community-Based Alternatives Among Blacks, Hispanics, and Whites (New York: Community Research Applications, 1980).

Examines black, white, Puerto Rican and Mexican American's information and attitudes about long-term care, community alternatives, and institutional care. Data collected from telephone interviews with 410 white, 399 black, 402 Mexican American, and 397 Puerto Rican respondents concerning demographic characteristics, attitudes toward and knowledge about availability, sources of reimbursement, referral sources, and actual service use in-home nurses, homemakers and nursing homes. The study did not substantiate a relationship between attitudes and knowledge about long-term care and actual service use among ethnic groups.

232. Kail, B.B. and Lukoff, I.F. "Differentials in the Treatment of Black Female Heroin Addicts." Drug and Alcohol Dependence 13 (1) (1984): 55-63.

The National Institute on Drug Abuse has placed special emphasis on meeting the unique requirements of female and minority addicts. Yet, few attempts have been made to delineate the needs of black female heroin addicts. Differentiation among black female addicts on the basis of treatment needs remains even more limited. This study of black men and women entering an inner-city methadone maintenance program attempts to fill that gap. Multiple discriminant analysis indicates that these women may not be one homogenous group. The typology developed for female respondents is quite similar to that developed for male respondents. Conclusion suggests that each type of black female addict has different treatment needs.

233. Kerr, G.R. et.al. "Supermarket Sales of High Sugar Products in Predominantly Black, Hispanic and White Census Tracts of Houston, Texas." American Journal of Clinical Nutrition 37 (4) (April 1983): 622-31.

Sales of 488 sweet foods and beverages by supermarkets located in predominantly black, Hispanic, and white census tracts of Houston, TX, were examined in relation to sales of a number of commodity foods. Mean sweet energy/commodity food sales ratios in black and Hispanic census tract supermarkets were 122% and 108%, respectively of those in white census tracts. Ethnic differences in sweet energy/commodity sales ratios were almost always statistically signficant (p less than 0.05), but variation within ethnic groups of supermarkets remained large, indicating that nonethnic factors also influenced the food purchase patterns. Supermarket sales records offer a relatively inexpensive source of data for comparative or longitudinal studies of community purchase of food products postulated to play a role in the development of nutrition-associated health problems. The major problems in interpreting the data result from a need to use ratios, and lack of a valid measure of the population consuming foods purchased.

234. Lairson, D., Lorimor, R. and Slater, C. "Estimates of the Demand for Health: Males in the Preretirement Years." Social Science and Medicine 19 (7) (1984): 741-47.

The demand for health is estimated for black and white males in the preretirement years using data from the first wave of 1966 National Longitudinal Survey of men aged 45-59. This survey includes direct measures of the wage rate and family assets. Findings for whites generally corroborate

Grossman's initial estimates of the demand for health. In contrast to whites, blacks show a much stronger wage effect and a significant positive effect of wife's education, with no other factors being significant. The issue of reverse causality between the wage and health is addressed via a simultaneous equations health-wage model. Contrary to what was expected, but consistent with previous findings, the structural model yielded an even larger wage effect.

39. Lee, A.S. and Lee, E.S. "The Health of Slaves and the Health of Freedmen: A Savannah Study." Phylon 38 (2) (June 1977): 170-80.

A study conducted in the nineteenth century by W. Duncan (Tabulated Mortuary Record of the City of Savannah, from January 1, 1854 to December 31, 1869. Savannah Morning News Steam-Power Press, 1870) offers a new source of data for demographic modeling of black populations. This was a period of repeated epidemics. Blacks were comparatively resistant to some of these, e.g., yellow fever, but not to others, e.g., smallpox or typhoid. Cancer and circulatory diseases were uncommon among both races. Suicide and homicide were unimportant among both races, but accidental death, especially by drowning, was quite common. Infant deaths were 25% higher among blacks, and deaths from fever were also more common, though low in both races. The health of blacks declined after the Civil War due to the lack of economic interest of whites in preserving the health of free black employees who had no resale value.

236. LeFlore, I.C. "Misconceptions Regarding Elective Plastic Surgery in the Black Patient." Journal of the National Medical Association 72 (10) (October 1980): 947-48.

Discusses some misconceptions in the medical and lay literature and by many surgeons regarding elective plastic surgery in black patients. Generally, it is felt that operating upon blacks is more hazardous and the results are unpredictable. Specifically, the problems of scarring, keloid formation, pigmentary changes, and psychological/ sociological adaptation are given as reasons for not performing elective surgery on blacks. Concludes that with very few exceptions elective plastic surgery can be performed on blacks in the same manner and using the same criteria of patient selection as for non-blacks, and with the same expected results.

237. Link, C.R., Long, S.H., Settle, R.F. "Access to Medical Care Under Medicaid: Differentials by Race." Journal of Health Politics, Policy, and Law 7 (2) (Summer 1982): 345-65.

Argues that previous evaluations of the Medicaid program have claimed that on average the eligible poor have enjoyed considerable gains in access, but that the benefits of Medicaid have not been shared equally by blacks and whites. Reexamines the differential access by race in the beginning of the program in 1969 and at maturity in 1976, allowing for socieconomic status, health status, and resource supply characteristics. Notes that while earlier evaluations overstated the extent of racial differentials, blacks who were chronically ill did have a significantly lower level of ambulatory care, both in and out of the South than whites. However, by 1976, blacks had clearly achieved equality with whites in ambulatory care use. The only statistically significant difference was in hospital utilization among Southern blacks in good health.

238. Linn, M.W., Hunter, K.I. and Linn, B.S. "Self-Assessed Health, Impairment and Disability in Anglo, Black and Cuban Elderly." Medical Care 18 (3) (March 1980): 282-88.

Self-assessed health and physician-rated impairment were compared for 174 Anglo, black, and Cuban elderly medical outpatients. Level of disability was also recorded by the interviewer. A minimal correlation was found between patient and physician-rated health. Self-assessed health and level of functioning were associated significantly in each of the 3 cultures. The patients perceived their health and functioned differed by culture, but impairment ratings of the physician did not discriminate among cultures. It seems likely that nonmedical factors may explain cultural differences in perception of health as well as how these perceptions influence ability to perform everyday activities of living. The patients' estimates of health appear to be an important factor in their overall health status, which physicians could use to augment their assessments of impairment. Since self-assessed health relates to level of functioning and to the way the elderly react to an illness, it can be seen as a useful component in evaluating health and predicting patient behavior.

239. Lloyd, S.M., Jr. and Johnson, D.G. "Practice Patterns of Black Physicians: Result of a Survey of Howard University College of Medicine Alumni." Journal of the National Medical Association 74 (2) (February 1982): 129-41.

Over 600 Howard University medical alumni of seven representative classes graduating from 1955 to 1975 were surveyed by questionnaires in 1975 and 1976. Replies of the 252 black respondents confirm that these graduates are providing substantial care to blacks, the economically disadvantaged, and in the inner city. Survey findings reaffirm the necessity to train more black physicians and to provide data on current and future practice patterns. Comparisons are made between the practice patterns of earlier (1955 to 1970) and later (1973 to 1975) black graduates. A general bibliography of publications relevant to the practice patterns of black physicians is included.

240. May, J.T. "A 19th Century Medical Care Program for Blacks: The Case of Freedman's Bureau." Anthropological Papers of the University of Alaska 46 (3) (July 1973): 160-71.

Admissions data from a southern, federally-sponsored hospital for blacks in the 1860's are used to pinpoint change in United States medical care policy. These changes, it is found, reflected the conflicts among sponsoring agencies (mainly the officials of the Union Army versus those of the Freedman's Bureau over authority and control, and had little to do with the actual needs of the target population. It is suggested that a resolution was achieved because federal officials and native whites sought a common end, the reestablishment of social order through a revival of the plantation economy. Attention is drawn, finally, to the value of historical analogues for the analysis of contemporary programs, such as the Office of Economic Opportunity. Beyond this is the larger question: To what extent may history be used to generate questions about contemporary phenomena?

241. McFalls, J.A. "The Impact of VD on the Fertility of the U.S. Black Population." Social Biology 20 (1) (March 1973): 2-19.

Beginning in the latter part of the 19th century, the birth rate of the United States black population began a steady decline, which continued until the late 1930's. Demographers have offered several possible explanations to account for this trend and for the rise in fertility that followed. One explanation, based on the premise that VD lowers fecundity, is that changes in VD prevalence were chiefly the rise in the birth rate in 1936. Arguments used to support this conclusion are examined and criticized. Key questions are given special attention: (1) Did VD increase enough between 1880 and 1936 to account for the observed fertility decline? It was found that the usual argument for a large increase, those centering on rudimentary VD prevalence data and inferences from urban/rural and childlessness differentials, proved faulty. Indeed, available information weighs against any great increase. (2) Was the sudden rise in the fertility around 1936 preceded by the effective control of VD in the black population? According to the VD fertility hypothesis, the black natality rise is explicable by a fall in VD prevalence resulting from the discovery and application of superior treatment methods and the simultaneous creation of government VD control programs. On the contrary, present data indicate that the sudden rise in fertility does not appear to have been preceded by the effective control of VD. Black fertility began to climb before the occurrence of substantial improvements in the quality and availability of treatment, and prior to meaningful reductions in VD prevalence. The control of VD was probably not the major factor in the upward fertility trend from 1936-1957. (3) What was the quantitative physiological impact of VD on fertility? It was found that VD, and syphilis in particular, has a milder physiologic impact on an individual's fecundity than had previously been thought. Despite unrealistically high assumptions of a 0 to 25% syphilis prevalence increase and a 0-50% gonorrhea prevalence increase, VD could have accounted for only about 20 of the observed natality change. Under lower and more realistic assumptions, this estimate would be substantially lower.

242. McShane, D. and Willenbring M.L. "Differences in Cerebral Asymmetries Related to Drinking History and Ethnicity: A Computerized Axial Tomography CAT Scan Study." Journal of Nervous and Mental Disease 172 (9) (September 1984): 529-32.

Normal computerized axial tomography scans of 179 American Indian, black and white subjects were examined for cerebral asymmetry patterns. Information concerning the drinking history of each subject was also obtained. Results indicated that alcohol use history was associated with differences in asymmetry patterns, above and beyond differences associated with ethnicity. In subjects without a history of alcohol use, more whites were more likely to have left asymmetry of both occipital length and width, as compared to American Indians and blacks. In subjects with a history of alcohol use, all subjects closely resembled one another, regardless of ethnicity. In the total sample, alcohol users were more likely to show greater right occipital width.

243. Medina, A.S. et.al. "Adolescent Health in Alameda County." Journal of Adolescent Health Care 2 (3) (March 1982): 175-82.

A cross-sectional study of 194 adolescents in Alameda County, California was performed to investigate health care behavior, personal adjustment, substance abuse, and medical and dental morbidity. A multivariate analysis of this sample using age, sex, ethnic group, and family type as independent variables was carried out.

Females were less likely than males to have a regular place for medical care, and youths belonging to single parent families were less likely than those from intact families. Older adolescents, blacks and Hispanics used hospitals and clinics more frequently, while whites used private physicians more frequently than did other ethnic groups. Also blacks and Hispanics were less likely to have received recent dental care than whites. Levels of substance abuse were comparable to national levels, and increased significantly with age. Though, overall medical morbidity was low, the study confirms previous findings of significant levels of dental decay particularly in black youth. A significant relation exists between medical care and medical morbidity. The study has potential implications for better preventive approaches to adolescent health care.

244. Meyer, L.D. et.al. "Prevalences of Anemia and Iron Deficiency Anemia in Black and White Women in the United States Estimated by Two Methods." American Journal of Public Health 73 (September 1983): 1042-47.

Prevalences of anemia were estimated by two methods for black and white nonpregnant women of childbearing age. One method defines the prevalence of anemia as the proportion of women whose hemoglobin values are shifted downward relative to a distribution of hemoglobin values of non-anemic women. Results produced by both methods suggest a higher prevalence of anemia in black than in white women. The distribution method is also used to estimate the contribution of iron deficiency to anemia. All anemia in white women and a high proportion of anemia in black women is associated with iron deficiency. The five variables related to anemia and examination attendance for black women were: presence of piped water; presence of hot and cold piped water; whether a language other than English was spoken at home; employment status; and whether the women worked outside the home.

245. Morgan, B.S. "Selected Correlates of White Nursing Students' Attitudes Toward Black American Patients." International Journal of Nursing Studies 20 (2) (1983): 109-21.

Discusses the relationships between white nursing students' attitudes toward black American patients and variables selected within a theoretical framework of prejudice which included socialization factors and personality-based factors. The variables selected were: authoritarianism and self-esteem (personality-based factors), parents' attitudes toward black Americans, peer attitudes toward black Americans, interracial contact and socioeconomic status (socialization factors). The study also examined the differences in the relationship among white nursing students enrolled in baccalaureate degree, associate degree and diploma nursing programs. The major findings of this study indicate that the socialization explanation of prejudice is more significant than the personality-based explanation.

246. Neighbors, H.W. "Professional Help Use Among Black Americans: Implications for Unmet Need." American Journal of Community Psychology (October 1984): 551-66.

Previous findings on black utilization have been largely obtained from racial comparison studies. Little attention has been paid to sociodemographic differences or the social psychological processes that affect help-seeking behavior within the black group. The present study analyzed data obtained from a national probability sample of the black population. A multidimensional contingency table analysis revealed that problems experienced by the lower income group were more serious than those experienced by the upper income group. Low-income respondents were also more likely to state that their personal distress was caused physical health problems. Income, however, was not related to the decision to seek professional help. The implications of these findings for understanding black illness behavior and the underutilization of services was discussed.

247. Neighbors, H.W. and Jackson, J.S. "The Use of Informal and Formal Help: Four Patterns of Illness Behavior in the Black Community." American Journal of Community Psychology 12 (6) (December 1984): 629-44.

Most studies of professionnal help use among black Americans fail to describe this group's relationship to blacks experiencing distress but not requesting professional help, and generally ignore the salience of informal social support processes. A more comprehensive understanding of black help-seeking behavior would come from an approach which describes both the users and nonuser of formal helping services, and examines the benefits derived from the interpersonal relationships that comprise black friend- and kin-based networks. These analyses focused on four patterns of informal and formal help use in the National Survey of Black Americans. The findings indicated that most people use informal help only, or they use informal and professional help together. In addition, gender, age, income, and problem-type were significantly related to the different patterns of illness behavior. The implications of these findings for help seeking in the black community were discussed.

248. Nurco, D.N. and Shaffer, J.W. "Types and Characteristics of Addicts in

the Community." Drug and Alcohol Dependence 9 (1) (February 1982): 43-78.

This study examines both the status and behavior of 230 white and 230 black male narcotic addicts. Following a presentation of antecedent behaviors and characteristics, an addict typology is developed based on illicit income, perception of adequacy of income to meet needs, and employment. The resulting six types are then described in terms of treatment experiences, criminality, social activities, and psychopathology. The discussion includes suggestions of a treatment perspective for each type.

249. Orr, S.T., Miller, C.A. and James, S.A. "Differences in Use of Health Services by Children According to Race: Relative Importance of Cultural and System-Related Factors." Medical Care 22 (9) (September 1984): 848-53.

Argues that black children do not make use of public health care or other health services in the same proportion as do white children, regardless of family income levels or financial status. Black children occupy a poorer health status than do white children in American society. Study focuses on system-related barriers to seeking health care among blacks and culturally-related patterns related to health and illness that account for observed differences in usage between blacks and whites. In comparing the use of health services by black and white children within a system of care that actively seeks to decrease "barriers" to access to care by black children, black and white children used health services in a similar fashion. Findings indicate system-related factors that assure equity of access to health services may be more important than client-related cultural factors.

250. Postell, W.D. The Health of Slaves on Southern Plantations (Baton Rouge, LA.: Louisiana State University Press, 1951).

Describes health care provided to slaves on plantations.

251. Pennici, E.A., "Stroke Data Bank Yields Scientific Information," Public Health Reports 98 (3) (May-June 1983): 300-1.

Summarizes the findings of the National Institute of Neurological and Communication Disorders and Stroke Data Bank. The first national computerized storehouse of information about stroke patients. It provides a pool of stroke related data that scientis can usets to detect patterns in the factors causing the disease and in evaluation and the effectiveness of treatment. Scientists have confirmed from this data that certain strokes are more common among blacks than whites. Scientists believe the incidence of stroke resulting from bleeding into the brain tissue itself is three

252. Pierce, R.O., Jr. "A Study of Bone Density in Black Women with Hip Fractures." Journal of the National Medical Association 74 (4) (April 1982): 325-27.

Fracture of the hip in black women is not a common injury. The cause of this decreased incidence is commonly stated to be the relative increase in density of the bones in black women as compared with whites. To test this hypothesis, the author studied the x-rays of 101 black women who had hip fractures, finding that there was a decrease in the mineral content of bone. Also examines the degree of kyphosis and found that this increased over the control group. This study does not refute the lower incidence of hip fracture in black women but simply points out that when these fractures do occur, they occur in osteopenic bone.

253. Peoples, M.D., Grimson, R.C. and Daughtry, G.L. "Evaluation of the Effects of the North Carolina Improved Pregnancy Outcome Project: Implications for State-Level Decision-Making." American Journal of Public Health 74 (6) (June 1984): 549-54.

Assesses the effects of the North Carolina Improved Pregnancy Outcome (IPO) Project on the use of prenatal care and incidence of low birth-weight among mostly black registrants. The IPO Project was started in 1976 to "improve maternal care and pregnancy outcomes in states which have contributed to the incidence of infant mortality." North Carolina selected a two county area that had a high rate of poverty, rurality and excessive rates of perinatal and infant mortality. One of the counties had no public or private maternity services while the other had few resources.

254. Rahbor, F. et.al. "Prenatal Care and Perinatal Mortality In a Black Population." Obstetrics and Gynecology 65 (3) (March 1985): 327-29.

Using three-year cumulative data relative to perinatal mortality, the study examines the relationship of prenatal care and birthweight to pregnancy outcome. The results support the hypothesis that links prenatal care to pregnancy outcome and the relationship between birth weight and pregnancy outcome is found to be strong. The study indicates that the knowledge of birth weight would reduce the number of errors in predicting the chances of survival of the newborn by 37.0%.

255. Relman, A.S. "Race and End-Stage Renal Disease." New England Journal of Medicine 306 (21) (1982): 1290-91.

Argues that end-stage renal disease (ESRD) develops more frequently in blacks than in whites in this country. Blacks constitute a disproportionately high percentage of the ESRD population-- 35% in one index and 29%

in another, as compared with about 12% in the national population. There is an increased rate among blacks in all age groups and both sexes, but the greatest relative risk is in the fourth decade, particularly in women. Studies show that much of the excess risk of uremia among blacks is due to an extraordinarily high rate of renal failure from hypertensive disease.

256. Robinson, J.C. "Racial Inequality and the Probability of Occupational--Related Injury or Illness" Milbank Memorial Fund Quarterly/Health and Society 62 (4) (Fall 1984): 567-590.

Begins with a consideration of the common issues at stake for public policy in the areas of public health and affirmative action. Discusses the evaluation of the measures of occupational hazards and measures which show that the concentration of black workers is in the most hazardous positions in the economy. The average black worker is found to be in an occupation 37 to 52 percent more likely to result in a serious injury or illness than the occupation of the average white worker. Forty-seven percent of the black workers report themselves as exposed to at least one hazard, compared to 37 percent of the whites. The race variable shows a strong influence on the likelihood of a black worker in a dangerous occupation. Advocates several strategies including strengthening E.E.O.C., Title VII and O.S.H.A.

257. Rostand, S.G. et.al. "Racial Differences in the Incidence of Treatment for End-Stage Renal Disease." New England Journal of Medicine 306 (21) (1982): 1276-79.

Analyzes patterns in a large urban county to determine the effects of age, race, sex, and cause of renal failure on rates of referral for treatment of ESRD. The study shows that in Jefferson County, Alabama, the average yearly rate at which new patients are referred for treatment of ESRD is approximately 9.1 per 100,000 population and that the apparent risk of ESRD is four times higher in blacks than in whites. Much of this difference is related to the finding that rates of hypertensive renal disease in blacks were 17 times rates in whites and that rates of diabetic kidney disease, chronic glomerulonephritis, and interstitial kidney disease were also much higher in blacks.

258. Salber, E., and Beza, A.G. "The Health Interview Survey and Minority Health." Medical Care 18 (3) (March 1980): 319-26.

Emphasizes the advantages and disadvantages of the National Center for Health Statistics Health Interview Surveys (HIS) when applied to the needs of ethnic minorities at the local level. The survey, while national in scope, samples a small number of minorities. As a result, a number of problems may arise. Recommends special national in-depth surveys of specific minority groups.

259. Sargent, M.B. "Summary of Market Research for Healthy Mothers, Healthy Babies Campaign." Public Health Reports 98 (4) (July/August 1983): 356-60.

The "Healthy Mothers, Healthy Babies" campaign was established in 1981. It grew out of a federal goal to improve U.S. infant and maternal mortality rates. U.S. infant mortality rates generally have declined over the last decade. However, the mortality rate for black infants remains almost twice as high as for white infants. As a result, Health and Human Services contracted with Juarez and Associates to conduct a market research study that would provide insights into the best ways to convey the needed health education to the target group of high risk mothers, of blacks and Hispanics. After the study, it was concluded that the physician was the most credible source of health information for the women despite the presumption expressed by most of them that the physician was often inaccessible and too busy to talk to them. However, in the public health clinic, nurses were the key contact.

260. Savitt, T. Medicine and Slavery: The Disease and Health Care of Blacks in Antebellum Virginia. (Urbana, IL.: University of Illinois Press 1978).

Focuses on Virginia from the Revolution to the Civil War. Provides an analysis of the kinds of diseases which afflicted the Old South's black conditions that existed at that time, and provides a historical perspective of the relationship between black health care and white society. Discusses how working conditions, clothing, cleanliness and food intake contributed to a slave's well-being or ill health.

261. Schneller, E. S. and Weiner, T. S. "The Black Physician's Assistant: Problems and Prospects". Journal of Medical Education 53 (August 1978): 661-66.

A report on a study of the social origins, attitudes, and anticipated practice settings of blacks and whites. Addresses comparisons on attitudes towards status, income stability, national health insurance and servicing the poor. Indicates that the black physician assistants have a higher desire to practice in ghetto areas than white physician assistants.

262. Schwartz, B. "Time, Patience and Black People: A Study of Temporal Access to Medical Care." Sociological Focus 11(1) (January 1978): 11-20.

Delay is an important feature of medical services because it is a barrier to convenient access. To be understood properly, however, it must be decomposed into its objective aspect, indexed by waiting time, and its subjective aspect, indexed by impatience. Data on 3,180 heads of household taken from a NORC national survey conducted in 1970 show that blacks wait longer for medical service than whites and are more dissatisfied per unit of delay. This finding is inconsistent with the popular assumption that blacks are less concerned than whites with time cost. Blacks' impatience and its adverse effects on utilization of medical services are greater in the radical and the more disadvantaged. These results stem not from specifically time-related values but from a diffuse negativity evoked by living under adverse social conditions which limit the extent to which increased patient satisfaction can be achieved by objective changes in the organization and distribution of medical services as such.

263. Sellers, R. V. "The Black Health Worker and the Black Health Consumer: New Roles for Both." American Journal of Public Health 60 (November 1970): 2154-70.

Describes the roles of the black health worker and the consumer in the delivery of health care.

264. Schutte, J. E. "Growth Standards for Blacks: Current Status." Journal of the National Medical Association 72 (10) (October 1980): 973-78.

Notes that growth standards specific to black boys and girls are necessary because genetically determined patterns of growth in black children are signficantly different from those of white children. Such standards have only recently become available and they need further refinement. The required improvements include: (1) adjusting the standards to reflect the range or variation in growth of middle-to-upper income blacks; (2) expanding the lower age range of the standards to include children of preschool age; and (3) periodic revaluation and reformulation of the standards to keep them current with secular increases in size and maturity among black children.

265. Shafer, S.Q. "The Contribution of Nonaneurysmal Intracranial Hemorrhage to Stroke Mortality in New York City Blacks." Strokes 4 (November/December 1973): 928-32.

Out of 527 unselected stroke patients (98% Blacks), 80 (17%) had nonaneurysmal intracranial hemmorrhages, with a fatility rate of 85%. Of 216 in-hospital deaths 37% were due to intracranial hemorrhages. In patients aged 65 and less, 52% of 90 fatal events were hemorrhagic. In patients below age 46, cerebral hemorrhage accounts for more deaths than infarction. The average age of black patients with fatal hemorrhage was 61 years. The following conclusions about spontaneous nonaneurysmal hemorrhage among blacks can be drawn: above age 45, it does not account for more deaths than infarction; it is not much more common or lethal in blacks than in whites; and it does not occur predominantly at earlier ages in blacks than in whites.

266. Shafer, S.Q. "Brain Infarction Risk Factors in Black New York Stroke Patients." Journal of Chronic Diseases 27 (January 1974): 127-33.

Points out that out of 527 stroke patients, 22 percent had a previous stroke; 57 percent had hypertension; 28 percent had diabetes mellitus; 24 percent had advanced heart disease; and 18 percent had none of these conditions. When the study divided patients by age, diabetes, and heart disease, previous strokes were more common in patients 65 and older. Hypertension was significantly less frequent. The Health Examination Survey estimated that 52 percent of blacks age 65-74 and 60 percent of those age 75-79 were hypertensive. However, for those studied prevalence of hypertension at ages 65-74 was 48 percent. It fell to 37 percent for ages 75 and over. In more aged patients, hypertension seemed to be less common than estimates note.

267. Shah, N.D. and McGhee, N. "Shift from Predominantly White to Predominantly Black Staff: A Retrospective Study Relating to Surgical Care." Journal of the National Medical Association 72 (7) (July 1980): 677-681.

Reports findings from 9-year study on hysterectomy patients at Southwest Community Hospital in Atlanta, Georgia. Indicates that a shift in hospital staff from predominantly white to predominantly black had no detrimental effect on quality of care. The study was conducted to test the hypothesis that hospitals with white staffs offered superior medical care. It also shows that the number of consultations increased with the influx of obstetrical/gynecological physicians. At the same time, there was approximately 90% positive correlation between clinical and pathological diagnoses with the influx of black obstetrical/ gynecological physicians to the staff.

268. Smoyak, S.A. "Nurse and Client Ethnicity and its Effects Upon Interaction" A Strategy for Change, American Nurses' Association, 1979): 46-71.

Presents an overview of culturally-centered ignorances among health professionals in relation to ethnic styles, patterns, and belief systems ("cultural traps") and identifies specific ways ethnicity can affect the nurse/client relationship in a "tolerance of difference" framework. General principles affecting the interaction of people of different backgrounds are highlighted and a specific paradigm for analyzing differing cultures is presented. Nurses as ethnic people of color and as collaborators with other nurses in providing quality health care is also discussed.

269. Snow, L.F. "Sorcerers, Saints and Charlatans: Black Folk Healers in Urban America." Culture, Medicine and Psychiatry 2(1) (March 1978): 69-106

> Black Americans who believe their illness has been caused by sorcery often believe their problems will not respond to orthodox medicine and may leave treatment to seek out folk healers. Healers believed to be able to cure sorcery are, however, seen ambivalently, since they are believed equally able to inflict harm as to cure it. The lack of information on these persons and their modes of treatment makes it dificult to assess their abilities. On the basis of contact with a number of such healers in an effort to learn more about them, it is concluded that some provide useful service to their clients, but that many use their reputations as manipulators of occult powers to extract money from the poor and qullible.

270. Spirey, G.H. and Radford, E.P. "Inner-City Housing and Respiratory Disease in Children: A Pilot Study." Archives of Environmental Health 34(1) (January/February 1979): 23-30.

> This cross-sectional pilot study, designed to examine problems and methodology of studies on the relationship of housing and health, focused on respiratory disease in inner-city black children in Baltimore. Public housing was contrasted to the older row private housing. History of illness, familial, and demographic characteristics were obtained by questionnaire, and a small subsample of children received physical examinations. The condition of the indoor environment was evaluated, and measurements of indoor temperature, volume, relative humidity, and carbon monoxide were made. Children in public housing had higher illness rates than those in private housing. Evidence of self-selection into housing type was found. Carbon monoxide levels were found to be greater inside than outside the homes. Preliminary analysis suqgests public-housing/private-housing classification is less important than other variables, including socioeconomic variables.

271. Steele, M.F. and Gallagher, M.L. "Lipid, Kilocalorie, and Selected Mineral Intakes of Rural Black Schoolgirls." American Journal of Public Health 75(11) (November 1985): 1323-24.

> Dietary intakes of nutrients implicated in cardiovascular disease were studied in 143 black females, age 9 years. Dietary recall interviews were conducted and data compared with recommendations of several authoritative groups. A majority of subjects reported intakes exceeding recommendations for total fat, saturated fat, and sodium; within recommendations for potassium and cholesterol; and below recommendations for kilocalories.

272. Termini, T.E., Biundo, J.J and Ziff, M.; The Rarity of Felty's Syndrome in Blacks." Arthritis and Rheumatism 22(9) (September 1979): 999.

Study was conducted at the Parkland Memorial Hospital located in Dallas, Texas, from 1964 through 1978, and at Charity Hospital, located in New Orleans, Louisiana from 1968 through 1978. Evidence is presented that Felty's Syndrome is very rare among black patients with rheumatoid arthritis.

273. Tolnay, S.E. "Trends in Total and Marital Fertility for Black Americans, 1886-1899." Demography 18(4) (November 1981): 443-63.

Total fertility rates and age-specific marital fertility rates are estimated for the urban and rural black populations during the last fourteen years of the nineteenth century. The data source is a 1-in-750 sample of households from the 1900 census manuscripts. The results show sharp differences in the levels of urban and rural reproduction as well as differences in the timing of the well-known black fertility transition. Calculation of Coale-Trussell m-values suggests that up to 1899, rural blacks were essentially a "natural fertility" population while urban residents apparently had a history of family limitation. These findings support the inference that at least some segments of the black population were practicing birth control before the turn of the twentieth century.

274. Tuckson, R. "The Black Physician and the Challenges of the 1980s." Journal of the National Medical Association 76(10) (October 1984): 977-80

Notes that the challenges which confront the black physician in the 1980s are numerous. As competition in the marketplace becomes progressively more intense, so do the pressures to organize into economically efficient, aggressive practice associations. The growth of health maintenance organizations, independent practice associations, and preferred-provider organizations will force the black physicians to concentrate on the business aspect of medicine as never before Cutbacks in public insurance programs and chronic black unemployment have already caused many black physicians to seek out new segments of the health care market. The imposition of diagnosis related groups as a basis for reimbursement has already raised serious concerns for black physicians and inner-city hospitals.

275. Vernon, S.W. et al. "Ethnic Status and Participation in Longitudinal Health Surveys." American Journal of Epidemiology 119(1) (1984): 99-113.

Ethnic differences in survey participation and their effects on self-reported physical and psychiatric health status measures were examined in a longitudinal health study in Alameda County, California. Blacks and Mexican-Americans were more likely than whites to refuse to participate in follow-up surveys and were more difficult to trace when the time interval between interviews was long. With the exception of age, demographic characteristics were not consistently associated with participation status, either across ethnic groups or across time periods. Self-reported psychiatric and physical health status were not statistically associated with participation status in any ethnic group for either time period, despite differential participation by ethnicity.

276. Wan, T.T. "Use of Health Services by the Elderly in Low-Income Communities." Milibank Memorial Fund Quarterly/Health and Society 60(1) (Winter 1982): 82-107.

Although it is generally assumed that there has been a narrowing of the gap in health care between poor and nonpoor families, the relative contributions of improved fiscal and geographic access are not well documented. Almost 2,000 elderly poor persons were studied to examine factors affecting their use of health services. A number of personal and structural problems are identified when cultural and ethnic backgrounds are considered.

277. Warnecke, R.B. and Graham, S. "Characteristics of Blacks Obtaining Papanicolaou Smears." Cancer 37(4) (April 1976) 2015-25.

An understanding of the characteristics of women who do not obtain cervical cytology may shed light on procedures which can be instituted by physicians and public health workers to increase use of screening. Of particular interest are women at high risk of cervical cancer. Interviewed a random sample of about 700 blacks living in central Buffalo census tracts in regard to their past use of pelvic examinations as well as circumstances surrounding such use or non-use. Employed only data on screening which was verified in records. Found that there was declining use with increasing age and lack of contact with physicians, clinics, or hospitals. The relationship between increasing use and increasing education was found to be a function of the fact that women with more education are likely to be younger. There was clear evidence that making such examinations part of the contact women have with physicians or hospitals for any purpose, including childbirth, would increase the proportions screened.

278. Westoff, C.F. and Ryder, N.B. "Contraceptive Practice Among Urban Blacks in the United States, 1965." The Milibank Memorial Fund Quarterly/Health and Society (April 1970): 215-39

Discusses the practice of contraception and family planning among the urban Black population of the United States with a special emphasis on their use of newer methods. Concludes that urban black women are more informed about the use of contraceptives than are black women in suburban or rural areas.

279. White, E.H. "Health and the Black Person: An Annotated Bibliography." American Journal of Nursing 74 (10) (October 1974): 1839-41.

An annotated listing of 69 readings from a broad range of literature reflecting the range of social, economic, and physiological conditions that affect the health and lives of black Americans. The readings were compiled by a nurse educator.

280. Wing, S. et.al. "The Black/White Mortality Crossover: Investigation in a Community-Based Study." Journal of Gerontology 40 (1) (January 1985): 78-84.

The black/white mortality crossover at about age 75, a result of lower white mortality rates at younger ages and lower black rates at the oldest ages, has been observed in U.S. vital statistics since 1900. Though a persistant observation in such data, its validity has been challenged by questions about census enumeration and age reporting on death certificates. Analyses of 20 years experience of all-cause mortality rates showed a community-based Evans County Study using a Weibull model of age specific mortality rates showed a statistically signficant black/white mortality crossover for both men (at age 73) and women (at age 85). The findings of a crossover in this longitudinally followed population is significant because the age reporting for both survivors and age at death for nonsurvivors were obtained in the study protocol and did not rely on age reporting either in census data or on the death certificate. Differences in the age and sex patterns of mortality between tow populations living in the same geographic region are relevant to questions about the etiology of the major age-related chronic diseases as well as to topics of current interest in health care policy.

281. Wolinsky, F.D. "Racial Differences in Illness Behavior." Journal of Community Health 8 (2) (Winter 1982): 87-101.

Using data on 359 white and 126 black respondents who were interviewed in their home as part of an omnibus health care study in a rural southern county during 1978, the illness behavior (i.e., dentist, physician, and hospital utilization measures) of black and whites are compared and contrasted. Zero-order racial differences in illness behavior disappeared after controlling for the predisposing, enabling, and need characteristics identified in R. Anderson's generic access model (A Behavioural Model of Families' Use of Health Services, Chicago: Center for Health Administration Studies, 1968). Further multivariate analysis, however, indicates that while there are no racial differences in illness behavior after the predisposing, enabling, and need characteristics of the individual are taken into consideration, there are significant differences between blacks and whites in the effects of these characteristics, at least in terms of discretionary health services utilization. This provides some support for recent speculation that blacks might respond differently than whites regarding the use of and access to health services because of separate cultural traditions.

282. Woolhandler, S. et.al. "Medical Care and Mortality: Racial Differences in Preventable Deaths." International Journal of Health Services 15 (1) (1985): 1-22.

Analyzes deaths of blacks and whites in Alameda County, California where previous studies have documented consistent racial inequalities in healh services. Classifies each death during June 1978 as due to preventable and manageable conditions or as "non-preventable." The total death rate for blacks 0-65 years of age exceeded that of whites by 58 percent. Rates of death due to preventable and manageable conditions for persons aged 0-65 years were 77 percent higher for blacks than for whites. More than one-third of the excess total death rate of blacks relative to whites could be explained by the excess of potentially preventable deaths. Findings suggest that inequalities in health services reinforce broader social inequalities and are in part responsible for disparities in health status. Improvements in the health and longevity of blacks must be achieved by improved access to existing medical, public health and other preventive measures.

5. Cancer

283. Agu, V.U., "Geographic Patterns of Multiple Myeloma: Racial and Industrial Correlates: State of Texas 1969-1979" National Cancer Institute Journal 63 (5) (October 1980): 1189-98.

Age adjusted mortality rates for multiple myeloma in Texas State Economic Areas (TSEA) were correlated with selected occupations. After control was made for the percentage of the population classified as black, the possible association between the age-adjusted mortality rate from multiple myeloma and percentage of the population in each TSEA employed in beauty shops, carpentry, and agricultural industry was significant. The findings emphasize the possible importance of race as a confounding variable in ecological analyses of environmental and industrial exposures associated with mortality due to multiple myeloma.

284. Alfred, L.J. et.al. "Release of Lymphotoxin By Control and Chemical Carcinogen Treated Lymphocyte Cultures Derived From From Black Healthy Subjects and Cancer Patients." Journal of the National Medical Association 74 (8) (August 1962): 775-86.

In an age-adjusted comparison with white men, black men have a significantly higher increase in esophageal and other types of cancer associated with environmental causes. The study measured certain cell-mediated immune reactions in cultured lymphocytes derived from black healthy subjects and cancer patients. The study also determined the levels of aryl hydrocarbon hydroxylase (AHH) induced in these lymphocytes.

285. Devesa, S.S. "Association of Breast Cancer and Cervical Cancer Incidences with Income and Education Among Whites and Blacks." National Cancer Institute Journal 65 (3) (September 1980): 515-28.

Data from the 1969-71 third National Cancer Survey were used to study the association of cancer incidence with income and education as indicated by census track of residence. Also considered was the effect of adjustment for differences, in socio-economic adjustment reduced by over half of the black and white differences in breast cancer rates, and education had a stronger effect than income. Conversely, the incidence of cancer of the cervix showed strong negative association with each of the two variables. The excess risk among black women was reduced by two thirds with socioeconomic adjustment, though rates remained significantly different.

286. Gaskin, H.S. et.al. "Multiple Primary Malignancies in Black Patients." Journal of the National Medical Association 73 (11) (December 1981): 1065-68.

Charts of 42 black patients with multiple malignant neoplasms were among 1,953 cancer patients selected for review during the period of 1959 through 1979. The incidence was 2.15%. Most patients were female and the breast was the most frequent initial primary carcinoma. With this relatively small number of cases, there was no consistent cluster of initial and second primaries about which to make inferences. In the absence of a regional registry of primary tumor incidence, no generalities could be obtained concerning a matched non-black population on the incidence of multiple primaries. However, comparison of this group could be made with data previously recorded.

287. Goldsen, A. et.al. Is There a Genetic Basis for the Differences in Cancer Incidence Between Afro-Americans and Euro-Americans?" Journal of the National Medical Association 73 (8) (August 1981): 701-6.

The data of the Third National Cancer Survey show, for many cancer types, large differences in cancer incidence between Euro-Americans and Afro-Americans. As in other racial studies, it is difficult to separate environmental and genetic factors. For the cancers which are more frequent among Afro-Americans, environmental factors seem to be primarily responsible. Among the cancers less frequent in Afro-Americans, there are some for which the racial differences have a genetic basis. Perhaps there is also a genetic basis for some of the racial differences in the incidence of malignant lymphomas and leukemias. For all these cancers, Afro-Americans are less susceptible.

288. Gregorio, D.I. et.al. "Delay, Stage of Disease, and Survival Among White and Black Women with Breast Cancer." American Journal of Public Health 73 (5) (May 1983): 590-93.

Delay in obtaining treatment, stage of disease at diagnosis, and 5-year survival were compared for 29 black and 156 white females treated for breast cancer at Roswell Park Memorial Institute between 1957 and 1965. No statistically significant differences were found between black and white patients in treatment delay, although a tendency for longer delay among blacks was noted. Findings showed black women delayed seeking treatment because they were less aware of breast cancer symptoms, more pessimistic about its curability, and less knowledgeable of screening procedures. Race had little effect on survival when delay, stage of disease, and age were controlled.

289. Haddy, T.B. "Cancer in Black Children." *American Journal of Pediatric Hematology/Oncology* 4 (3) (1982): 285-92.

A review of the literature indicates that black children in the U.S. have a lower overall incidence of cancer and are less prone to leukemia and certain solid tumors, including neuroblastoma, rhabdomyosarcoma, Ewing's sarcoma, testicular tumors, liver tumors, and malignant melanoma, than are white children. Black children with acute lymphoblastic leukemia and retinoblastoma, but not with neuroblastoma, Wilms' tumor, and rhabdomyosarcoma have poorer survival rates than white children. Socioeconomic status appears to be an important reason for the discrepant outlook, but genetic differences may also play a role. Consideration of these issues will assist in planning appropriate treatment regimens.

290. Hall, H. "Cancer and Blacks: The Second-Leading Cause of Death" *Urban League Review* 9 (2) (Winter 1985/86): 26-31.

Discussion focuses on cancer as the second leading cause of death for black Americans. The direct effects on cancer initiation show three risk factors: alcohol use, tobacco use and occupational exposure to carcinogens. The indirect effects include high fat diet and stress. The direct effects on cancer progression include the relationship between distress and coping with progression. The final category is the indirect effects on cancer progression which for blacks is the delay in seeking medical diagnosis and medical treatment. Socio-economic status and poverty also fall within this final category as well as geographic location.

291. Kovi, J. "Gastric Cancer In American Negroes." *Cancer* 34 (July 1974): 765-70.

A study at Howard University Hospital of gastric cancer of 110 black males and 40 females.

292. Matsuoka, L.Y. and Schquer, P.K. "Basal Cell Carcinoma in Black Patients." *Journal of the Medicine Academy of Dermatology* 4 (6) (June 1981): 670-72.

Fourteen cases of basal cell carcinoma occurring in North American black patients are reviewed. The majority of the lesions were asymptomatic, hyperpigmented, translucent nodules and were diagnosed as being basal cell carcinomas prior to biopsy. All of the lesions, except one, arose in the sun-exposed areas of the head, neck and hands, indicating that basal cell carcinoma in blacks, as in whites, is related to exposure to ultraviolet light. Microscopic examination revealed changes characteristic of basal cell carcinoma. The response to therapy was good and there appeared to be no histologic or clinical differences in the basal cell carcinomas that arise in black and white patients.

293. Michielutte, R. and Diseker, R.A. "Racial Differences in Knowledge of Cancer: A Pilot Study." Social Science and Medicine 16 (3) (1982): 245-52.

   Examined the reported sources of information on cancer and the level of cancer knowledge for a sample of black and white adults. Black respondents had significantly less knowledge and the relationship between race and cancer knowledge persisted even when controlling for education, sex, and age. Possible reasons for the observed differences include (a) the tendency for blacks to obtain information on cancer from television and radio, while whites rely more on printed materials, (b) differences in the quality of education received by black and white adults, and (c) a possible lack of motivation on the part of black responsdents to acquire knowledge of cancer due to lower access to medical care. Intervention programs designed to provide all blacks with information about cancer should take into account the preferred sources of information, and should be oriented toward reducing the barriers to taking action related to prevention and early detection as well as increasing perceptions of the benefits of taking such action.

294. Miller, J.M. and Chapman, T.W. "Reviewing Cancer in American Blacks: A Baltimore Study." Journal of the National Medical Association 73 (2) (February 1981): 127-32.

   Rates for the incidence and mortality of cancer have greatly increased in black Americans as they have been assimilated into Western culture. In cancer of certain types, prevalence is greater and survival is poorer in blacks than in whites. Moreover, a significant increase among blacks is plainly evident in a comparison of statistics of 30 or more years ago and the present. There are many apparent causes for this change, and perhaps one factor is the mixing of genetic backgrounds to produce a single population. Heightened rates may be stemmed, however, by directing greater attention to prevention of cancer by elimination of carcinogens from the environment.

295. Miller, W.J. and Cooper, R. "Rising Lung Cancer Death Rates Among Black Men: The Importance of Occupation and Social Class." Journal of the National Medical Association 74 (3) (March 1982): 253-58.

   From 1950 to 1977 the age-adjusted cancer death rates for nonwhite men in the U.S. rose an astonishing 63.2%, while rates for white men increased 22.2% and fell slightly for women of both races. The bulk of this increase can be accounted for by cancer of the lung. As a serious health problem that is increasing in severity, cancer in blacks deserves close attention and definitive action. Discussion focuses on basic epidemiological relationships in the origin of this epidemic, particularly in regard to the relative importance of occupation, cigarette smoking, and social class.

296. Pottern, L.M. et.al. "Esophageal Cancer Among Black Men in Washington, D.C.: Alcohol, Tobacco and Other Risk Factors." <u>Journal of the National Cancer Institute</u> 67 (4) (October 1981): 777-83.

A case-control study involving interviews with the next of kin or close friends of 120 black males who recently died of esophageal cancer and 250 similarly aged black males who died of other causes was undertaken to discover reasons for the exceptionally high mortality from this cancer in Washington, D.C.. The age-adjusted annual death rate in Washington, D.C. for nonwhite males, 1970-71, was 28.6/100,000; far higher than the national rate of 12.4/100,000 and the rates in other metropolitan areas of the country. The major factor responsible for the excess was alcoholic beverage consumption, with an estimated 81% of the esophageal cancers attributed to its use; high use of alcoholic beverages was also found among the controls. The relative risk (RR) of esophageal cancer associated with use of alcoholic beverages was 6.4 (95% confidence interval = 2.5., 16.4). The RR increased with amount of ethanol consumed and was highest among drinkers of hard liquor, although the risk was also elevated among consumers of wine and/or beer only. The RR associated with cigarette smoking was 1.9 (1.0. 3.5) when controls with smoking-related causes of death were excluded by declined to 1.5(0.7.3.0) when adjusted for ethanol consumption. Significant differences of approximately twofold were found between low and high levels of a) consumption of fresh or frozen meat and fish, fruits and vegetables, and dairy products and eggs and b) relative weight (wt/ht2). The inverse trends with these general measures of nutritional status were not explained by alcoholic beverage consumption or socioeconomic status as measured by educational level.

297. Pressior, R. and Chung, E.B. "Granular Cell Tumor in Black Patients." <u>Journal of the National Medical Association</u> 72 (12) (December 1980): 1171-75.

A 12-year review of granular cell tumors at Howard University Hospital is reported. Sixty-one cases were studied (56 patients). A female preponderance was clearly established and multicentricity of lesions constituted a higher percentage than previously reported in other series. Malignant transformation was not found. Electron microscopic studies tended to support the Schwan cell origin theory for the tumor but no conclusion could be drawn as to whether the lesion is neoplastic, degenerative, or metabolic in nature.

298. Ries, L.G. "Cancer Patient Survival: Surveillance, Epidemiology, and End Results Program, 1973-79," National Cancer Institute Journal 70 (4) (April 1983): 693-707.

> Data from the Surveillance, Epidemiology, and End Results (SEER) Program of the National Cancer Institute were used in the evaluation of cancer patients survival experiences for almost 10 percent of the U.S. population. The report contains actual (life table) survival analysis on 386,263 patients with primary cancer diagnosed in 1973-79 from nine SEER areas. Regarding race, the largest difference was seen in cancer of the corpus uteri: For white males, the site with highest survival rate was the bladder (72%), whereas for black males, the highest survival rate was found by those with cancer of the prostate gland (54%). For white females, the highest rate was for cancer of the corpus uteri (87%); for black females the highest rate was for cancer of the cervic uteri (61%).

299. Rochat, R.W. "Pap Smear Screening: Has it Lowered Cervical Mortality Among Black Americans?" Phylon 38 (December 1977): 429-47.

> Discusses cervical cancer mortality trend for black Americans, factors which may have affected this trend, and the accuracy of cervical cancer diagnoses. Cervical cancer mortality among black Americans has declined, first among younger women and later among older women. There is evidence to support the hypothesis that the mortality decline was due to a change in inherent risks among recent birth cohorts. The most influential cause of the mortality decline was probably surgical removal of the cervix. There is a expected lag time of 10-15 years between hysterectomy and a prevented death from cervical cancer. Cervical cancer screening was probably not a major cause of the early mortality decline, but may be an important factor in the slightly accelerated decline.

300. Rogers, E.L. Goldkind, L. and Goldkind, S.F. "Increasing Frequency of Esophageal Cancer Among Black Male Veterans." Cancer 49 (3) (February 1982): 610-17.

> Between the years of 1975 and 1979, the frequency of diagnosis of esophageal cancer has doubled at the Baltimore VA Medical Center due to a rapid increase of esophageal cancer among black males. This increase was not related to increased yearly hospital admission rates, percentage of black patients admitted yearly, or increased use of the hospital for chronic disease processes. Detailed chart review and comparison with consecutive medical

admissions as controls revealed heavy alcohol use and urbanization to be risk factors experienced more frequently by black than white male verterans. A serious question needs to be quickly answered: Does the rise of esophageal cancer at the Baltimore VAMC reflect a rise among black males only in Baltimore or does it reflect a rise nationwide among black males with a history of previous employment in the armed forces?

301. Rosen, T. et.al. "Bowen's Disease in Blacks." Journal of the American Academy of Dermatology 7 (9) (1982): 364-68.

It is generally accepted that solar irradiation plays a major role in the development of many cutaneous neoplasms. Thus, tumors such as Bowen's disease are common in light-skinned, sun-sensitive individuals. Among Caucasians, these epidermal tumors arise more often in individuals with fair skin color than in those with swarthy skin. Therefore, the foregoing neoplasms are relatively rare in blacks. The occurrence of Bowen's disease in blacks has been only infrequently noted in the literature. However, the authors believe this phenomenon to be more frequent than heretofore recognized. Seven such cases are presented to illustrate clinical and histologic features. Arsenic exposure is implicated in some instances.

302. Smith, R.J. "Melanoma in Black Patients." Journal of the National Medical Association 74 (4) (April 1982): 377-80.

Melanoma (skin cancer) in black patients is uncommon but not rare. Discusses six cases seen in one general surgeon's practice in Arkansas during a 14-year period. A review of the current literature regarding melanoma in blacks is provided. Characteristically, melanoma in blacks is found on the soles of the feet, palms of the hands, or mucous membranes. The tumor has a deadly potential unless it is treated at an early stage. Four of the patients discussed have died of metastatic disease. A public health program is needed to make physicians and the public aware of the incidence and location of this tumor.

303. Steinhorn, S.C. "Characteristics of Colon Cancer Patients Reported in Population-Based Tumor Registries and Comprehensive Cancer Centers" National Cancer Institute Journal 70 (4) (April 1983): 629-34.

The characteristics of colon cancer tumors diagnosed in patients seen at hospitals participating in the national Cancer institute's Surveillance, Epidemiology, and Education Results (STEER) Program and at Comprehensive Cancer Centers (CCC's) are compared. Ninty percent of the colon tumors in the STEER program occurred among whites, compared to 84.2 percent in the CCC's. Tumors for black patients accounted for 68.3 percent of tumors among nonwhites in the STEER program, but for 97.7 percent of the tumors among the nonwhites in the CCC's. This may reflect the fact that many CCC's are located in older predominantly black urban areas in the east, whereas the STEER registries cover areas in the west and southwest, with high concentrations of Hispanics and whites.

304. White, J.E. "Cancer Differences in the Black and Caucasian Population." Phylon 38 (September 1977): 297-314.

Compares cancer death in the black and white populations from 1949 to 1967. Concludes that cancer deaths are increasing two times faster for blacks and higher cancer mortality is more pronounced among the black male. Some of the factors considered as causes of the increased black cancer mortality rates are higher exposure to carcinogens, dietary habits, inferior socio-economic conditions, greater incidence of predisposing diseases, lower cure rates, errors in the census enumeration, less accurate death certificates and genetic differences. Among the cancers occurring more frequently in blacks are those of the esophagus, stomach liver, biliary passages, pancreas, prostrate, cervix, and urinary bladder. One reason for the increase in cancer mortality in blacks is that they recieve poorer care with diagnosis made in later stages of cancer when treatment is less effective.

305. Young, J.L., Jr. "Incidence of Cancer in the United States Blacks." Cancer Research 35 (November 1975): 3523-36.

Incidence rates for the black population shows black males have the highest rate among the major races and black females had the lowest rates. It is suggested that high rates among black males can be explained by census underenumeration. While there was considerable underenumeration of black males, aged 20 to 54, there was an overenumeration of black males aged 65 and over. High rates among black males cannot be explained on the basis of denominators that were too low. An analysis of survey data by socioeconomic status will be undertaken in hope of understanding the black/white differences in cancer diagnosis.

306. Young, J.L., Jr. "Cancer Patient Survival Among Ethnic Groups in the U.S." National Cancer Institute Journal 73 (2) (August 1984): 341-52.

Data from the Surveillance, Epidemiolgy, and End Results program of the National Cancer Institute were used in the evaluation of cancer patient survival for eight racial-ethnic groups in the U.S. population. Rates were uniformly low among each group for cancer of the esophagus, liver, and pancreas. Survival rates for Hispanics were almost identical to those for whites. The white survival rate was 48 percent while the black rate was 36 percent.

6. Political/Social Issues

307. Ahmed, P.I. and Coelho, G.V. Toward a New Definition of Health (New York: Plenum Press, 1979): Chapters 6, 11, and 12

Although minorities are mentioned throughout the text, health care for blacks is discussed primarily in Chapter 12 and to some extent in Chapters 6 and 11. Higher incidence of certain health problems among some minorities in the United States is attributed to dietary or cultural habits, and the book identifies that a reordering of society's institutions, priorities, and values is needed. Blacks are said to avoid private physicians and dentists and to rely heavily on over-the-counter medicines. The authors do acknowledge, however, that most of the sub-culture research is out of date due partially to changes in availability of health care providers among minorities during the 1960's and 1970's. Observes that it is apparent that minorities' reasons for avoidance of medical care may be economically and not culturally biased.

308. Barber, J.B. and Sinnette, C.H. "Presidential Politics and Minority Health." Journal of the National Medical Association 76 (10) (October 1984): 969-71.

During a presidential campaign, health care issues receive little attention. Such issues as the rising cost of health care, inaccessibility of medical care, maldistribution of health care providers, and Medicare bankruptcy, and a fragmented health care system elicited few meaningful comments or constructive proposals from the 1984 presidential candidates or their parties.

309. Bullough, V.L. and Bullough B. Health Care for the Other Americans. (New York: Appleton-Century-Crofts, 1982): Chapter 3.

This chapter argues that the health problems faced by the black community remain monumental. The chapter reveals how these problems can be understood by examining the past history of black Americans because this past has left its mark on today. Three variables seem most important in explaining the fact that mortality and morbidity rates are higher for blacks. They are poverty, discrimination, and the social-psychological barriers. These variables tend to prevent blacks from using health services that are available. All three of these variables interact and reinforce one another, just as poor health care interacts with and reinforces other problems faced by the black community.

310. Cates, W., Jr. "Legal Abortion: Are Black Women Healthier Because of It?" Phylon 38 (3) (September 1977): 267-81.

In the United States, despite relatively greater disapprovals of abortion by black women, legal abortion is used by them at approximately twice the rate of their white counterparts. Moreover, the disproportionate use of legal abortion by black women has been increasing since the 1973 Supreme Court decision making legal abortion available locally. Because legal abortions are safer than other alternatives facing black women with unwanted pregnancies, e.g. illegal abortions or term births, they have a positive effect on their health, as demonstrated through reduced levels of morbidity and mortality from pregnancy and childbirth. Moreover, legal abortion has probably contributed to the reduction of unwanted births to married black women, reducing such births to the same level as that of white women. For these reasons, it is apparent that black women have shared in the health benefits accompanying increased availability of legal abortion, probably to an even greater extent than white women.

311. Clark, H.W. "How Relevant is the Free Clinic Movement to Black People." Journal of Social Issues 30 (1) (1974): 67-72.

A philosophical and practical look at the free clinic as a significant alternative to the lack of health care in black communities. Serious questions are raised about setting up, in a haphazard way, discrete clinics to meet the needs of the community. The concept of health care delivery, the use of federal funds, and the need for the power structure to maintain its political machination base are indicated. It is suggested that as medical schools, the government, and agencies coopt free clinics, they will be less and less "free" unless the struggle becomes a national and unified one.

312. Cooper R. et.al "Racism, Society and Disease: An Exploration of the Social and Biological Mechanisms of Differential Mortality." International Journal of Health Services 11 (3) (1981): 389-414.

Racial differential in mortality provide important insight into the nature of mass disease in capitalist society. Not only are they sizable in magnitude, they are consistent for multiple causes of death and appear to evolve in response to social development. The relationships among social factors and the biological and physical agents of disease can be identified through racial contrasts and a pattern of causation which applies to both the minority and majority populations described. Furthermore, the impact of exploitation as the primary disease-mediating factor under capitalist social relations can be estimated. This paper attempts to combine an analysis of bio-medical mechanisms with Marxist social theory in comprehensive framework for the study of the social origins of racial differentials.

313. Curtis, J.L. "Civil Rights in Medicine." Journal of Public Health Policy 1 (2) (June 1980): 110-20.

Notes that the current effort to improve the status of civil rights for underrepresented minority groups in the U.S. proceeds on two fronts: equalizing minority access to health career education and training opportunity and equalizing minority access to health care. Inadequate attention has been given to both measures to remove continuing racial barriers to both of these avenues to health care opportunity. Presents the need for specifically race-conscious policies and actions to remove the ingrained racial injustice still to be found in the American health care and health educational systems.

314. Creighton, H. "Law for the Nurse Manager: Hospital Guilty of Racial Discrimination." Nursing Management 14 (3) (March 1983): 20-21.

Reviews the case of racial discrimination in employment involving M.D. Anderson Hospital located in Houston, Texas.

315. Davidson, A.T. and Coleman, A.H. "Health Care and the Law: The Legal Status of Physicians on hospital Staffs." Journal of the National Medical Association 75 (1) (January 1983): 87-8.

Addresses the legal status of physicians on hospital staffs, with a concentration on black and other minority physicians. Explains the problem of the courts trying to decide if a physician is an employee or an independent contractor in relation to his/her services in dealing with a hospital.

316. Davidson, A.T. and Coleman, A.H. "Health Care and the Law: Legal Options in Securing Hospital Appointments." Journal of the National Medical Association 75 (3) (March 1983): 318-20.

Examines the legal options available to black physicians in securing hospital appointments.

317. Dutton, D.B. Socioeconomic Status and Children's Health" Medical Care 23 (2) (February 1985): 142-53.

Explores the U-Shaped relation between family income and three common children's health problems: ear disease, hearing loss, and vision problems. Data are based on clinical examinations of 1,063 black children of varying income levels, conducted in 1971 in Washington, D.C.. The three health problems displayed a U-shaped relation to income, although only ear disease and vision problems displayed this pattern in national data.

318. Feagin, J.R. and Feagin C.B. Discrimination American Style (Englewood Cliffs, N.J.: Prentice Hall, Inc., 1978) Chapter 5: 135-38.

Inequality in medical facilities has a significant impact on the health and well-being of minority persons. The negative result is evident in data which show sharply higher death and disease rates for nonwhite Americans.

319. Fiori, F.B., "Bureau of Health Facilities Increasing Responsibilities in Assuring Medical Care for the Needy and Services without Discrimination." Public Health Reports 95 (2) (March/April 1980): 164-73.

Addresses the mission and responsibility of the Bureau of Health Facilities in implementing a portion of the Hill-Burton Act for providing for uncompensated care for the poor and with community services that facilities agreed to provide in exchange for financial aid received from Federal Government. The Bureau has inherited the responsibility for monitoring programs and facilities which received direct and guaranteed loan under Title VI of Public Health Service Act. Overall, the Bureau has adopted the responsibility for assuring medical care to those unable to afford care by enforcing compliance with the laws and regulations established to ensure suitable medical care is provided under the law to the underserved.

320. Gould, K.H. "Black Women in Double Jeopardy: A Perspective on Birth Control." Health and Social Worker 9 (2) (1984): 96-105.

Some segments of the black community consider birth control programs a disguised form of genocide. This historical analysis reviews how black women were discriminated against by forces in two social movements championing women's rights and demonstrates why some black people may associate family planning services with racism and efforts to eliminate their race. Explores the thesis that attitudes relating family planning to racism and genocide have historical roots in birth control and the women's movements and that black women were the targets of racist and anti-working-class attitudes prevalent among the conservative forces in both movements.

321. Gray, L.C., "The Geographic and Functional Distribution of Black Physicians: Some Research and Policy Considerations." American Journal of Public Health 67 (6) (June 1977): 519-26.

Reflects on the need for geographic and functional distribution of physicians studies to include the race of the physicians as a study variable. Reviews existing data on the geographic and functional specialty, source of income, and major professional activity distributing black physicians as compared to all physicians. Relates major issues in health manpower research and equity in medical career opportunity.

322. Harrison, I.E. and Harrison, D.S. "The Black Family Experience and Health Behavior" in Health And The Family: A Medical-Sociological Analysis. Charles O. Crawford (ed). (New York: Macmillan Co., 1971), Chapter 9.

It is most important that health practitioners, administrators, and any other persons responsible for decisions in the organization and provision of health care learn to understand the black family experience, look for strengths in the black community, and not view the life of black persons as a complex of pathologies which must be treated as such. Concludes that once health officials and the black community bridge this mental barrier, they will have achieved an important and necessary breakthrough in providing black families with quality health care.

323. Orque, Modesta S., "Health Care and Minority Clients." Nursing Outlook 24 (May 1976): 313-16.

Identifies a professional training course for nursing students at University of California at SF. The course is intended to increase knowledge of pyschological and cultural effects that affect health care of minorities and sharpen skills in relating to ethnic minority clients. Identifies different ethnic groups, the differences in groups, and provides a comparison of the problems and needs for specialized care and treatment based on cultural and ethnic background of recipient of care

324. Jackson, R.K. "The Effects of the Organizational Setting on Ethnic Nurses and Clients," A Strategy for Change, American Nurses Association (St. Louis, Missouri: American Nurses' Association, 1979): 72-102.

Beginning with an overview of health care delivery issues -- political, social, medical, ethical -- describes the generalized structure and ideals for public health care in America (availability, accessibility, appropriateness, adequateness, affordibility, acceptability, and accountability) Emphasizes the external socio-political factors affecting public health care and the lack of equity in provision of health care to minority clients and the opportunities afforded minority nurses and other health professionals. Difficulties in professional nursing for nurses of color are divided into five categories: (1) differing cultural backgrounds that affect language, goals, values, and perceptions; (2) low-to middle status work within a rigid, status-conscious, hierarchial institutional setting; (3) differing conceptions of self and expectations of others; (4) institutional facism and sexism; and (5) inequitable distribution of organizational resources that assures them of the least amount. Examines organizational settings, ethnicity and the effects upon the nurse/client relationship; delineates data and assesses and gives direction to the future data collection for change. Identifies and describes major components of health care delivery arrangements and discusses the nature of their organization and its impact on ethnic nurses and clients of color. Reviews the findings of a survey of 47 hospitals in the U.S. regarding decision making at the highest level and type of minority representation during the process. Offers practical suggestions and strategies for change.

325. Kiple, Kenneth F. Another Dimension to the Black Diaspora: Diet, Disease, and Racism (Cambridge: The Press Syndicate of the University of Cambridge, 1981).

Traces black health and disease through the periods of slavery and emancipation to present. Argues that the black health crisis will not be resolved by the education of the American medical profession. Rather, its failure in delivering proper medical care to blacks must be viewed within a larger context of public ignorance and policy-making indifference, neither of which is free of racism.

326. Lythcott, G.I. "Discrimination, Poverty, Described as Co-repressors of Health Care," U.S. Medical 16 (11) (June 1, 1980): 22.

Illustrates examples of discrimination in medical care. Specifically notes that major causes are related to the lack of representation of poor, elderly and inadequate representation of minorities on state health boards. Addresses national health care and the fact that it may not be the solution because of the lack of adequate facilities in areas where it is needed. Cites the need for encouraging more minority students to serve in primary health care field and the need for use of civil rights legislation to be used in a preventive manner instead of to alleviate discrimination.

327. Miles, M.E. The Effect of Social Class on the Degree of Congruence Between the Self Assessed and Rates Evaluated Functional Health Status of the Noninstitutionalized Aged Black Female. (North Central Sociological Association, 1982).

In old age, why do some people with significant physical problems continue to function while some give up? What are the determininants of such behavior? In the summer of 1981 a study was conducted in Cleveland, Ohio to determine if social class might be one determinant of perceptions of functional adequacy. Using church rolls, a sample of 100 noninstitutionalized black women, aged 65+ was selected to be interviewed. It was hypothesized that the higher the social class, the more realistic the perception would be. Realistic perception was defined as congruence between self-assessment and the rater evaluation of functional activities. It was further assumed that social class would continue to be a strong determinant when such variables as health knowledge, geographic location in childhood,, willingness to assume the sick role, chronicity, present assessment of health and current utilization of health services were introduced. The hypotheses were not substantiated; there was very little variability among the respondents. None were in the congruence or pessimistic ranges. The majority of the women were realistic about their functional health status. This supported the assumption that as a coping mechanism the black females of those generations had to perceive themselves as well in order work and survive.

328. National League for Nursing, National League for Nursing Position Statement on Nursing's Responsibility to Minorities and Disadvantaged Groups. (New York: National League for Nursing Publications, 1979).

Position statement promotes the ideal that people merit the removal of all legal and social barriers that deprive racial and minority groups of opportunities essential to their full participation in society without loss of respect for the cultural heritage of people or of tolerance for individual differences. In nursing education, emphasis is placed on the recruitment of members of minorities and on the development of remedial programs to enhance the probability of success in a nursing career. In nursing services, the National League of Nursing recognizes the urgency of meeting the special needs and problems of racial and ethnic minorities and the economically and socially disadvantaged without compromise in quality of care and with respect for the client's cultural, social and economical background. Specific steps for the attainment of goals in these two areas, nursing education and nursing services, are outlined. Nursing education objectives include suggestions for recruitment, admission, retention, curriculum, and faculty. Nursing services objectives include suggestions for nursing care methodology, job recruitment, selection of staff, retention of staff and promotion of staff.

329. Ory, H.W. et.al. "Mortality Among Young Black Women Using Contraceptives." Journal of the American Medical Association 251 (8) (February 1984): 1044-48.

Analyzes the mortality rates for young, black inner-city women, who used one of four methods of contraception--oral contraceptives, depomedroxyprogesterone acetate, intrauterine (contraceptive) devices, and barrier methods. The subjects were 30,580 15- to 44-year-old women who enrolled at a family planning clinic between 1967 and 1972 and who were observed by monitoring death certificates through the end of 1977. Forty percent of the 218 deaths observed were from accidents and violence. Use of this family planning clinic greatly reduced the risk of death from childbearing. Only two deaths were associated with pregnancy and childbirth, compared with the 24 deaths expected. Overall, users of the four methods died at similar low rates. Given that this study involves considerable loss to follow-up, possible acute effects of contraceptives (eg. infections or thrombosis) are more accurately estimated than possible long-term effects (eg. cancer).

330. Rice, H. and Payne, L. "Health Issues For The Eighties" in the National Urban League The State of Black America, 1981 (N.Y.: National Urban League, Inc.): 119-151.

Observes that from the mid-sixties through the mid-to-late seventies, there were over 75 separate items of federal legislation directed towards providing greater access to basic health services for the disadvantaged. The philosophy underlying this legislation was that there was a connection between health and poverty and if access to health services were improved, then this would lead to an improved health status which would help the poor to break out of their poverty. In most cases the legislation called for 1000 Neighborhood Family care centers serving 25 million low income persons. However, only 160 were funded serving only one and one-half million persons. Similarly, the 27 million people who live in a primar care manpower shortage area are minorities, even though projections show there will soon be a surplus of physicians. The number of minorities working in the health professions usually are employed in the lower paying secondary sectors. For blacks, 53 percent work as nursing aides, orderlies, and attendants as compared to only 22 percent of the whites. Only 3 percent of blacks serve in the higher paying jobs as compared to 20 percent of whites. There was also a major difference between whites and blacks who were without health insurance in 1977. Only 11.7 percent of whites compared to 18 percent of minorities were uninsured. Another major problem is the 40 percent of black children who still live in poverty in 1977. Finally, the authors provide items for a future health agenda: support of financially distressed hospitals; adoption of a child health program; support for health professions in education and training; opposition to across-the-board cuts in Medicaid; and government support of upward mobility programs.

331. Rice, M.F. and Jones, W. Jr. "Black Health Care in an Era of Retrenchment Politics" in M.F. Rice and Woodrow Jones Jr., Contemporary Public Policy Perspectives and Black Americans. (Westport, CT.: Greenwood Press, 1984): Chapter 10.

This chapter examines health status disparities in the Black community and observes that inadequate health care has always been a problem in the black community. The block grant system initiated by the Reagan Administration will not solve the crisis of health care in the black community particularly in the areas of health planning and health manpower distribution. Budget cuts will not provide the planning and personnel necessary tomak e conditions better. Additional funding for health care is needed to develop a comprehensive plan to provide a fair and equitable distribution of health care in the black community. The problems of black health care are directly related to the conditions of the black community. The combination of poverty, unemployment, and poor housing produce health conditions that are far inferior to those of the white population.

332. Rice, M.F. and Jones, W. Jr. "Health Care, Public Policy and the Courts: Black Health Status as a Civil Rights Issue." Health Policy 5 (1985): 207-21.

In the U.S. serious differences in health status between blacks and whites continue to exist. Black Americans are less healthy and receive less health care than white Americans. This discrimination is examined as a civil rights issue with a focus on both the policy and judicial perspectives of the application of Title VI of the Civil Rights Act of 1964 and the implementative effects of the Hill-Burton Act of 1946. The application, compliance, and enforcement of civil rights to health care is complicated by the captivity process involving Federal agencies, by corporate medical rights emphasizing a business approach to health care, and by a liberal, pluralistic political arena in which certain influential groups prevail over others. In order for black health status to improve in the U.S., blacks must continue to utilize the judicial system to seek redress of health care inequities. Second, blacks must utilize their demonstrated political power to demand better treatment from the medical establishment.

333. Ruffin, J.E. "Changing Perspectives on Ethnicity and Health": A Strategy for Change. American Nurses' Association (St. Louis, Missouri: American Nurses' Association, 1979): 1-45.

Overview of nursing professionalism and nursing services relative to ethnic and culturally disadvantaged groups. Includes principles for nursing care: (1) ethnicity is inseparable from American political realities; (2) racism in health care is slow to disappear; (3) progress in scientific research and professional work on issues in ethnicity in health care is slowed by both "cultural racism" and "institutional racism." Poverty and its effects upon ethnic and cultural minorities are emphasized, particularly the medical profession's inability or lack of dedication for separation of "social class" and medicine. Sociological, anthropological, and medical contributions to ethnic-centered health care are discussed as health status and needs, environmental factors and physical health, life expectancy, morbidity rates, nutritional deficiencies, environmental factors and mental health, and cultural differences among minority groups -- Asian Americans, Black Americans, Native Americans, Spanish Origin Americans, and White Americans. Outlines genetically influenced disorders among minority groups (congenital malformation, polydactyl, sickle cell disease, cancer(s), lupous erythematosus, tuberculosis, hypertensive heart disease and hyertension, uterine "fibroids", lactose intolerance, gout, acatalasia). Includes specific recommendation for improvement to the present system.

334. Schatzkin, A. et.al. "Antiracism and Level of Health Services: A Sociomedical Hypothesis." Journal of the National Medical Association 76 (4) (May 1984): 381-86.

Discusses the theory that antiracist efforts in health sector lead to an expansion of services and opportunities for minority and majority populations. Provides an evaluation of civil rights movements and their effect, results of antiracist movements, discussion relative to success in improved care due to movement.

335. Seham, M. Blacks and American Medical care (Minneapolis: The University of Minnesota Press, 1973).

Discusses the right to health and argues it is rhetoric rather than reality and that our emphasis on materialism plays an important role in health care in the United States. Presents the pattern of discrimination against blacks in American medicine and medical care to blacks in a large midwestern city. Observes that racism must also be considered as a public health problem and racism has its most profound effect on the mental and physical health of the minority groups. Diagnosis of the plight of blacks in American medicine is that today's medical system consists of twentieth-century technology shackled with nineteenth-century sociology. Details efforts that have been made to reverse the discrimination in black health care, offers some suggestions for future actions, and emphasizes the urgency of the need.

336. Southern Christian Leadership Conference, Crisis in Health Care for Black and Poor Americans (Atlanta, GA.: Southern Christian Leadership Conference, July 1984).

Report on the health status and health problems of blacks and other poor. Based on hearings conducted by the Southern Christian Leadership Conference in eleven cities to "take the pulse of those who were most likely to be adversely impacted by the recent changes in the responsiveness of the health care industry to recent tampering, turmoil and torment created by those of 'less than noble stripe' interfering with an industry whose functioning is usually characterized as humanitarian, compassionate, conscientious, caring and dedicated."

337. Stokes, L., "Search for Better Health Care in the Black Community." Journal of the National Medical Association 70 (1) (October 1978): 749-52.

Identifies factors influencing health status of the black community and points out a major need for consumer education to improve health status of black community. Also addresses federal health care programs and the rising demands which have occured since medicare and medicaid. Discusses drug abuse in the black community and program inequities in federal programs and the contribution of Congressional Black Caucus to areas of drug abuse, health, and communications.

338. Thompson, T., "Health and Social Policy Issues of Significance to Blacks in the "New Federalism." Journal of the National Medical Association 65 (5) (1973): 422-25.

Health and social policy issues of significance to blacks in the "New Federalism" are discussed. The New Federalism concept purports to return government to the people, but the people are the state and local governments which have tended to deprive blacks of the political and economic resources required for survival. Some of the issues of racism and discrimination in the American health insitutions discussed are discrimination in medical staff appointments, and the training and hiring of black and minority administrators in voluntary and teaching hospitals. Fewer minority doctors and dentists are being graduated from medical and dental schools, in spite of the fact that the federal government has appropriated large sums for health manpower training. The conclusion is that there is a need for a National Black Health Manpower policy which is concerned with the quantity and quality of the black health workers. There is a need also for a coalition of all black professional groups and consumer groups concerned with the health of blacks.

339. Turner, T. "Health Care Issues in Southern Rural Black America" Urban League Review 9 (2) (Winter 1985/86): 47-51.

Rural areas in the U.S., particularly in the southern U.S., are plagued by persistent health-care problems. This is especially true for the disproportionate number of blacks residing in rural areas of most southern states. The lack of black physicians, lack of health facilities, and access problems seem to be the major problems for blacks in rural areas.

340. Weaver, J.L. National Health Policy and the Underserved: Ethnic Minorities, and the Elderly (St. Louis, Missouri: C.V. Mosby Company, 1976).

Discusses the issues and problems in health care, public and private, involving minority and ethnic clients. After an overview of social and cultural class issues normally associated with minority health care, the author focuses upon the "community" approach to program and services evaluation and potential for health care policy and program reforms. Minorities discussed include Japanese, Philipinos, blacks, low income whites, elderly and Mexican-Americans within the U.S.. Information and statistics are those obtained from a Southern California study paralleling census tract data for the same area. Topics of discussion include information about health care providers; social patterns and health care problems of minority groups; poverty and health in blacks and whites; the public's opinion of national health insurance; health policy making; and common bases of health care problems.

341. Weaver, J.L. and Garrett, S.D. "Sexism and Racism in the American Health Care Industry: A Comparative Analysis." International Journal of Health Services 8 (4) (1978): 677-703.

By drawing on a wide range of material, a picture emerges of extensive abuse, discrimination, and exploitation of women and ethnic minorities at the hands of the American health industry. The number of minorities and women in professional schools and among the "elite" strata of the industry remain dispropor- tionately low. As patients, they receive often inferior, insensitive treatment. Overall, there is a remarkable similarity in the situation of women and minorities, a condition which reflects the perva- siveness of racism and sexism in American institutions and ideologies.

342. White, E.H. "Giving Health Care to Minority Patients." Nursing Clinics of North America

12 (1) (March 1977): 27-40.

> Health care is usually thought of as a basic right of each individual. This so-called basic right is denied to many mainly because of their economic situation and the color of their skin. There is a need for more blacks, Indians, Mexican-Americans Puerto Ricans, and Asians in the health care field. The numbers are low and the training process slow. Time is needed to prepare ethnic people of color. Since whites deliver most health services, they must become sensitive to the traditions of minorities. Nursing schools are beginning to include cultural differences in nursing curriculums, but the majority of the nurses who practice are not aware of and are not sensitive to the needs of nonwhite patients. Nurses must become personally involved in eradicating the injustice in health care. As Marie Branch states, there must be "personal reeducation." When this occurs, health care to the minority client will improve.

343. Winn, M. "Market Freedom/Competition, Health Care and the Black Community" Urban League Review 9 (2) (Winter 1985-86): 59-63.

> Argues that a reduction in public funds and support for health care will have an adverse impact on blacks. A competitive health system will increase the death rate.

7. Sickle Cell Anemia

344. Abramson, H., Bertles, J.F. and Wethers, D.L. Sickle Cell Disease: Diagnosis, Management, Education, and Research (St. Louis: The C.V. Mosby Company, 1973).

> Discusses the sickle cell disease as a worldwide problem and traces the clinical factors of this inherited malady of blacks through a child's early years, adulthood, and old age. Several chapters are devoted to the technical and clinical details, but they also give attention to the laboratory encounters with affected patients, management of sickle cell clinics, screening and counseling of patients, and various other problems and legal issues.

345. Adler, F.H. Textbook of Ophthalmology (Philadelphia: W.B. Saunders Company, 1962): Chapter 21.

> The chapter identifies symptoms for the ophthalmologist to observe and subsequently suspect and test for the presence of the sickle cell disease.

346. Alavi, J.B. "Sickle cell Anemia: Pathophysiology and Treatment." Medical Clinics of North America 6 (3) (May 1984): 545-56.

> Briefly outlines the pathophysiology and current therapy of the many problems encountered in treating the sickle cell patient. The emphasis is on sickle cell anemia (homozygous SS disease), although the pathophysiology of sickle-hemoglobin C or sickle-thalassemia is quite similar.

347. Buchanan, G.R. et.al. "Bacterial Infection and D Splenic Reticuloendothelial Function in Children with Hemoglobin SC Disease." Pediatrics 72 (1) (July 1983): 93-98.

> The type and frequency of invasive bacterial diseases were examined in 51 children with SC disease followed for 370 person-years, and splenic function was assessed in 31 patients by quantitation of pitted erythrocytes. Seven serious bacterial infections occurred in four of the patients, five due to Streptococcus pneumoniae and two to Haemophilus influenza. A

primary focus of infection was present in all episodes, none of which proved fatal. Although 30 episodes of pneumonia and chest syndrome occurred in 20 of the patients, a bacterial etiology was proven in only three instances. Splenic function was usually impaired, with a mean pit amount of 7.1% + 8.2% (range 0% to 22.9%). This is significantly greater than normal, but less than pit counts in patients with SS disease or asplenic subjects. Children with SC disease may have a greater risk of bacterial infection than normal children, but their infection rate is not nearly as high as that in patients with SS disease.

348. Chang, H. et.al. "Comparative Evaluation of Fifteen Anti-Sickling Agents." Blood 61 (4) (April 1983): 693-704.

Fifteen compounds reported to be inhibitors of gelation or sickling were studied by standard methods. These tests included (1) the determination of the solubility of deoxyhemoglobin S or C, (2) evaluation of sickling in whole SS affinity of hemoglobin and blood at various pO_2s, (3) measurement of the oxygen affinity of hemoglobin and blood, and (4) examination of red cell indices and morphology. Among the 4 noncovalent agents tested, butylurea was the most potent inhibitor of gelatin and sickling in vitro; however, relatively high concentrations were required compared to the covalent agents. In the latter group, bis- (3.5 dibromosalicyl)-fumarate, nitrogen mustard, and dimethyladipimidate were especially effective inhibitors of gelation and/or sickling. All of these compounds require further development before they can be considered for clinical use.

349. Charache, S. "Treatment of Sickle Cell Anemia." Annual Review of Medicine 32 (1981): 195-206.

Controlled trials of treatment for sickle cell anemia have shown only that proposed therapies were ineffective. Discusses one important mode of therapy for sickle cell anemia - "attention to complications that can be treated."

350. Cincinatti Comprehensive Sickle Cell Center, Evaluation of Patients with Sickle Cell Disease (Cincinnati, OH.: Cincinnati Comprehensive Sickle Cell Center, 1978).

A comprehensive technical manual designed to guide housestaff in their evaluation and treatment of patients with sickle cell disease.

351. Fabian, R.H. and Peters, B.H. "Neurological Complications of Hemoglobin SC Disease." Archives of Neurology 41 (3) (March 1984): 289-92.

The records of 68 patients with hemoglobin SC disease and 68 age- and sex-matched control patients were previewed for neurological problems.

A significant increase in retinopathy, stupor/coma, and seizures was noted in the hemoglobin SC group. Hemiplegia, noted in two young patients, was probably also secondary to hemoglobin SC disease. Hemoglobin SC disease may often go unrecognized as a cause of stupor and coma in older patients without other obvious manifestations of a sickling hemoglobinopathy. Factors known to precipitate sickling crisis and the associated neurological complications should be avoided, especially in patients undergoing surgery or parturition.

352. Farfel, M.R. and Holtzman, N.A. "Education, Consent, and Counseling in Sickle Cell Screening Programs: Report of a Survey." American Journal of Public Health 74 (4) (April 1984): 373-75.

In 1980, surveyed screening facilities to determine the extent of sickle cell screening and to assess compliance with Maryland regulations. Approximately 52,000 persons were screened per year in Maryland by local health departments, hospitals, primary care centers, correctional facilities, and units dedicated entirely to screening. Thirteen thousand persons were screened without informed consent. Many facilities were deficient in providing education and counseling as well as in obtaining informed consent. Units dedicated entirely to screening were compliant with the state regulations.

353. Ferrer, T.L. "Counseling Patients with Genetic Abnormalities." Nursing Clinics of North America 10 (2) (June 1975): 293-305.

Discusses counseling in regard to two major genetic deviations: glucose 6 phosphate dehydrogenase (G-6-PD) deficiency and the more common hemoglobinopathies. The impressions relating to genetic counseling are based on two years of personal experience among a low-income population of pregnant women in the Special Obstetrics Hematology clinics of the Maternal and Infant Care Project at Grady Memorial Hospital, Atlanta, Georgia. Genetic counseling is part of the multidisciplinary care routinely offered to pregnant women. Eighty-five per cent of the women in these special clinics are black. Criteria for referral to the Obstetrics Hematology clinics include the presence of any hematologic abnormality. Offers specific background for providing counseling care and presents information on the defects, awareness of the scope of patient responses, and trends in patient behavior.

354. Finelli, P.F. "Sickle Cell Trait and Transient Monocular Blindness." American Journal of Ophthalmology 81 (6) (June 1976): 850-51.

Five episodes of transient monocular blindness during a six-month period occurred in a 42-year-old black man who had sickle cell trait. Other than the hemoglobin abnormality no cause for the transient monocular blindness was determined.

355. Hick, E.J., Miller, G.D. and Horton, R. "Prevalence of Sickle Cell Trait and HBC-Trait in Blacks from Low Socioeconomic Conditions." American Journal of Public Health 68 (11) (November 1978): 1135-37.

Did not observe age or sex differentials in the prevalence of sickle cell or HBC-traits in black males or females of low socioeconomic status. When data were compared to those of others, found no evidence for a socioeconomic differential in the prevalence of these traits.

356. Jones, R.L. et.al. "Integrating the Teaching of Sickle Cell Anemia into the Curriculum of the Cincinnati Public School System." Journal of the National Medical Association 72 (2) (February 1980): 105-9.

In an effort to determine the impact of one aspect of the Cincinnati Comprehensive Sickle Cell Center's education program, a study of the level of knowledge of sickle cell facts by elementary and secondary school students in the Cincinnati public school system was conducted. An underlying assumption of this study was that a specially adapted sickle cell teaching curriculum in conjunction with in-service training for science teachers by sickle cell education staff was effective and practical. The study provided support for this assumption and has important implications for educating the general public about sickle cell disease and sickle cell trait.

357. Lang, F. "Sickle Cell and the Pill: Birth Control Pills Dangerous to Black Women." Ramparts (February 1972): 14-16.

Notes that birth control pills may be dangerous to a large number of black women. Suggests that women with sickle cell anemia or the sickle cell trait may be likely to develop blood clots if they take oral contraceptives. Before prescribing oral contraceptives, black women must be given a simple, inexpensive test to determine if they have the sickle cell trait. Nor are blacks warned that oral contraceptives in combination with the sickle cell trait may make them more susceptible to stroke or heart attack or other blood clots. Also discusses the causes of sickle cell and problems which might be caused during pregnancy and finally concludes by discussing some other hazards oral contraceptives may pose to black women.

358. Linde, S.M. Sickle Cell: A Complete Guide to Prevention and Treatment (New York: Pavilion Publishing Company, Inc., 1972).

Provides an overview of the disease and discusses who is susceptible as well as how the trait is passed on. Screening tests are discussed and their importance is stressed. Who should obtain the tests and when is discussed, as well as the kinds of tests that are given. The Jamaica Hospital Sickle Cell Clinic in New York City is examined as to the care given and what patients can expect. Caring for children with the disease is covered as are prevention tactics. Frequency of the sickle cell crisis, its causes, hospitals--are delineated. Also covers experimental treatments.

359. Matthews, M.S. "Cholelithiasis: A Differential Diagnosis in Abdominal 'Crisis' of Sickle Cell Anemia." Journal of the National Medical Association 73 (3) (March 1981): 271-73.

Observes that most recent literature on sickle cell disease has shown gallstones to be present in approximately 67% of affected patients. There is adequate evidence to urge all physicians to be aware of the contributions of gall bladder disease to the abdominal symptoms of sickle cell anemia. Frequently, because it is difficult to distinguish between the painful "crisis" and gall bladder disease, the latter diagnosis is not considered. Argues that investigative procedures of the gall bladder in all patients with sickle cell disease and abdominal crisis should be performed. If gallstones are present, elective cholecystectomy in the adequately prepared patient is recommended.

360. McFarlane, J. "Sickle Cell Disorders." American Journal of Nursing 77 (December 1977): 1948-54.

Sickle cell trait, sickle cell anemia, Sickle C, and sickle thalassemia are all caused by abnormal hemoglobin molecules that can produce deformity in red blood cells. Explains the differences and tells what information patients need.

361. Mears, G.J. et.al. "Alpha-Thalassemia Is Related to Prolonged Survival in Sickle Cell Anemia." Blood 62 (2) (August 1983): 286-90.

Determined the frequency of deletional a-thalassemia in black populations in the USA and Africa that harbor sickle cell anemia. In normals, the frequency of the chromosome bearing a deletion of one of the two normal x gene loci, designated (-a), ranged from 0.12 to 0.16 and in sickle trait subjects, the frequency was significantly greater and ranged from 0.18 to 0.20. Analysis demonstrated that the greater frequency in the last group was primarily a result of an increased number of subjects with a-thalassemia trait (also called homozygous a-thalassemia-2. In addition, the frequency of the (-a) chromosome was to increase progressively with age, supporting the hypothesis that a-thalassemia is favorable to the survival of subjects with sickle cell anemia. Thus, individuals who inherit a-thalassemia and sickle cell anemia may represent a subgroup of patients with a longer life expectancy.

362. National Center for Education in Maternal and Child Health, Sickle Cell: A Selected Resource Bibliography (Washington, D.C.: National Center for Education in Maternal and Child Health, October 1985).

A resource bibliography listing of educational and informational material on both sickle cell disease and trait. Also includes sources of printed and audiovisual materials.

363. Reing, A.B. "Learning and Behavioral Correlates in Learning-Disabled Pupils Prone to Heterozygous Thalassemia and Sicklemia." Journal of Genetic Psychology 127 (December 1975): 305-16.

The pilot study was designed to vindicate planning for large-scale detection and management of two parallel genetic blood disorders occurring in large numbers of Mediterranean and black Americans; the heterozygous minor traits of thalassemia (Cooley's anemia) and sicklemia (sickle-cell anemia). Referred pupils (N=191) matched on schools, age, and learning difficulties associated with learning disabilities were compared as to presumed ethnic origin (n Mediterranean = 80; n black = 64; n "others": = 47) and incidence of trait-related learning and behavioral characteristics. Group mean differences on the study's criteria were found to be significant. Both minor-trait prone groups equally indicated the associative effects, while the control group without tradition-predispositions showed a nonsignificant relationship, thus supporting the hypotheses and the need for large-scale research.

364. Samuels-Reid, J.H et.al. "Contraceptive Practices and Reproductive Patterns in Sickle Cell Disease." Journal of the National Medical Association 76 (9) (September 1984): 879-83.

A questionnaire was administered to 52 female subjects with sickle cell disease and to 80 control subjects. Questions were asked concerning contraceptive habits, reproductive patterns, and sexual activity. Findings indicate that sexual activity differed significantly for the two groups; only 38% of the females in the sickle cell group reported sexual activity compared with 81% of the females in the control group. Contraception was used less frequently by the sickle cell group. The sickle cell patients experienced more miscarriages and premature births. There was a greater percentage of cesarean sections in these patients (46%) compared with controls (18%).

365. Savitt, T. "The Invisible Malady: SIckle Cell Anemia in America, 1910-1970." Journal of the National Medical Association 73 (8) (August 1981): 739-46.

Observes that although articles have appeared on the history of sickle cell anemia in the U.S., none have dealt with the dissemination of information from the scientific community to the public. After the first case was documented in Chicago in 1910, more than 60 years passed before this important but racially oriented disease reached the public forum. Researchers in 1969 found that less than 20% of blacks knew about sickle cell anemia. Describes the major events in the history of sickle cell anemia and explains why it has not been publicized.

366. Schmidt, R.M. "Hemoglobinopathy Screening." American Journal of Public Health 64 (8) (August 1974): 799-804.

A unified public health approach toward screening for sickle cell disease and trait is presented. The goals of abnormal hemoglobin screening programs and their diagnostic, educational, and counseling requirements are discussed.

367. Schwartz, A.L. and Helfgott, M.A. "The Incidence of Sickle Trait in Blacks Requiring Filtering Surgery." Annals of Ophthalmology 9 (8) (August 1977): 957-59.

Open-angle glaucoma in the blacks is generally thought to be a more malignant disease than in whites in terms of response to therapy and subsequent visual loss. An increased incidence of unsuspected sickle trait and undetected sickling may have contributed to these patients' optic nerve ischemia, progressive field loss and need for surgery. A hemoglobin electrophoresis was done on 40 black patients who required filtering surgery for uncontrolled open-angle glaucoma. Only 2 of the 40 patients (5%) had sickle cell trait as determined by the hemoglobin electrophoresis. In a matched group of 40 controls, only 3 patients (7.5%) had incidence of sickle trait in black patients requiring filtering surgery.

368. Scott, R.B. (ed.) Advances in the Pathophysiology, Diagnosis, and Treatment of Sickle Cell Disease (New York: Alan R. Liss, Inc., 1982).

Presentation of current research in pathophysiology and applications of current knowledge in diagnosis, prenatal diagnosis and treatment of sickle cell disease and sickle-beta thalassemia.

369. Uy, C.G. and Scott, R.B. Guidelines for Care of Patients with Sickle Cell Disease (Washington, D.C.: Howard University Center for Sickle Cell Disease, 1978).

> Manual for physicians providing services to patients with sickle cell disease. Outlines emergency room, in-patient clinic care, management procedures, screening, reproduction and psychosocial and counseling services.

370. Walters, Ida et.al. "Complications of Sickle Cell Disease." Clinics of North American, Symposium on Sickle Cell Disease 18 (1) (March 1983): 139-84.

> Discusses the complications of sickle cell disease. Major complications of sickle cell disease can be categorized into acute events, chronic events, or health-related events that require added medical attention. Acute events include painful episodes, acute chest syndrome, right upper quadrant syndrome, skeletal and joint events, hand-foot syndrome, cerebrovascular accidents, aplastic episodes, sequestration renal complications, aseptic necrosis, and ocular complications. Health related events include delayed growth and development, delayed sexual maturation, pregnancy, surgery and anesthesia, and transfusions.

371. Whitten, C.F. et.al. "Sickle Cell Trait Counseling: Evaluation of Counselors and Counselees." American Journal of Human Genetics 33 (5) (1981): 802-16.

> In this study, information about both counselee and counselor performance was obtained from taped recordings of 193 structured counseling sessions with persons diagnosed as having sickle cell trait. The data provide evidence that: (1) lay persons can understand essential sickle cell information; (2) trained lay persons using a structured format can transmit successfully sickle cell information; (3) only education and age among counselee characteristics studied, were related to successful learning; (4) the evaluation of information transfer in counseling programs cannot be limited to counselees; comprehension but must also consider other variables such as counselor performance and curriculum content; (5) a reduction in negative feelings associated with a diagnosis of sickle cell trait is an immediate effect of counseling; and (6) audio-taping of counseling sessions is client-acceptable and useful for evaluation, quality control, and counselor training.

Appendix: Black Health Organizations

1. Association of Black Psychologists
   P. O. Box 2929
   Washington, D.C. 20013

2. Black Caucus of Health Workers
   c/o Albert M. Head
   MIC/PRESCAD
   1200 Sixth Street
   Suite M-146 Michigan Plaza
   Detroit, MI 48226

3. Black Psychiatrists of America
   P. O. Box 370659
   Decatur, GA

4. Health Braintrust
   Congressional Black Caucus Foundation
   1004 Pennsylvania Avenue, SE
   Washington, D.C. 20525

5. National Association for Sickle Cell Disease
   4221 Wilshire Blvd, Suite 360
   Los Angeles, CA 90010

6. National Association of Health Service Executives
   840 North Lakeshore Dr. 8 West
   Chicago, IL 60611

7. National Association of Medical Minority Educators
   Division of Student Affairs
   Medical College of Georgia
   Augusta, GA 30912

8. National Black Alcoholism Council
   417 South Dearborn Street
   Suite 1000
   Chicago, IL 60606

9. National Black Child Development Institute
   1463 Rhode Island Ave, NW
   Washington, D.C. 20005

10. National Black Health Planners' Association
    P. O. Box 28203
    Washington, D.C. 20005

11. National Black Nurses' Association
    P. O. Box 18358
    Boston, MA 02118

12. National Caucus and Center on Black Aged
    1424 K. Street, NW
    Suite 500
    Washington, D.C. 20005

13. National Dental Association
    5506 Connecticut Ave, NW
    Suites 24-25
    Washington, D.C. 20015

14. National Medical Association
    1012 Tenth Street, NW
    Washington, D.C. 20001

15. National Pharmaceutical
    Association
    2300 4th Street, NW
    Washington, D.C. 20059

16. National Society of Allied
    Health
    P. O. Box 494
    Howard University
    Washington, D.C. 20059

Author Index

A

Abramson, H. 344
Adebimpe, V.R. 40, 41, 42
Adler, F.H. 345
Agu, V.U. 283
Ahmed, P.I. 307
Ahmed, S.S. 1
Alavi, J.B. 346
Alfred, L.J. 284
Anderson, R. 171
Andreopoulos, S. 135
Argeriou, M. 136
Armstrong, H. 198
Ausubel, D.P. 43

B

Baker, F.M. 44
Balla, D.A. 90
Barbara, O.A. 45
Barber, J.B. 137, 308
Bell, C.C. 46, 47, 48, 49
Benjamin, M. 199
Benjamin, R. 199
Berenson, G.S. 2
Bertles, J.F. 344
Beza, A.G. 255
Biundo, J.J. 272
Blake, J.H. 200
Blum, J.D. 100
Blumenstein, B.A. 3
Boone, L.R. 50
Boyer, E. 201
Bowser, B.P. 51
Bradshaw, W.H. 52
Brancato, R. 1
Brandt, E.N. 138
Brantley, T. 53
Brayboy, T.L. 114
Brink, S.G. 139
Brunswick, A.F. 202, 203
Buchanan, G.R. 347
Bullough, B. 309
Bullough, V.L. 309
Bush, James A. 54

C

Caetano, D.F. 211
Caetano, R. 204
Callan, A. 148
Callender, C.O. 205
Cannon, M.S. 55
Carriera, R.P. 87
Carroll, J.R. 56
Carter, J.H. 57, 58, 59, 60, 61, 62, 63, 95, 123, 141
Cartwright, S. 206
Cates, W., Jr. 310
Cavenar, J.O., Jr. 140
Centerwall, B.S. 207
Chang, H. 348
Chapman, T.W. 294
Charache, S. 349
Chee, P. 208
Chung, E.B. 297
Cincinnati Comprehensive Sickle Cell Center 350
Clark, H.W. 311
Clifford, P. 144, 179
Coelho, G.V. 307
Coleman, A.H. 315, 316
Collins, J.E. 4
Cooper, R. 146, 295, 312
Cornely, P.B. 147
Cowan, M.A. 65, 129
Craig, T.J. 66, 67
Creighton, H. 314
Crood, T.H. 110
Cruckshank, J.K. 5
Curry, C.L. 6
Curtis, J.L. 313
Cutter, G. 31

D

Daughtry, G.L. 253
Davidson, A.T. 315, 316
Davidson, D.W. 210
Davis, W.E. 63, 129
Decker, D.L. 211
Devesa, S.S. 285

AUTHOR INDEX

Diseker, R.A.   293
Douglas, M.D.   3
Driscoll, D.P.   212
Durant, R.H.   213
Dutton, D.B.   317

E

Edgerton, R.B.   88
Edwards, G.F.   214
Edwards, L.N.   215
Egbert, L.D.   216
Eng, E.   148

F

Fabian, R.H.   351
Fabrega, H., Jr.   149
Farfel, M.R.   352
Farmer, M.E.   217
Faulkner, A.O.   70
Feagin, C.B.   318
Feagin, J.R.   318
Felaer, E.   150
Ferrer, T.L.   353
Finelli, P.F.   354
Fiori, F.B.   319
Flaherty, J.A.   71
Flaskerud, J.H.   72
Freedman, E.W.   218
Fried, J.   42
Friedman, E.   151
Fulwood, R.   34
Futrell, M.F.   219

G

Gaines, V.P.   220
Gallagher, M.L.   271
Galloway, N.O.   221
Garfinkel, L.   7
Gam, S.M.   222
Garrett, S.D.   341
Gartside, P.S.   8
Gary, L.E.   73, 74
Gaskin, H.S.   286
Gayles, J.N., Jr.   152
Gibbs, J.T.   75
Gluek, C.J.   11

Goldenberg, R.L.   153
Goldkind, L.   300
Goldkind, S.F.   300
Goldsen, A.   287
Goldstein, G.   224
Gordon, M.   154
Gordon, W.C.   225
Gould, K.H.   320
Graham, S.   277
Gray, B.A.   79, 80, 81
Gray, L.C.   321
Green, P.D.   63
Greene, R.L.   128
Greene, S.   226
Gregorio, D.I.   288
Griffith, E.H.   155
Grimson, R.C.   253
Grossman, M.   215
Gundlach, R.H.   118

H

Haddy, T.B.   289
Hadley, J.   156
Haigh, N.Z.   12, 227
Hall, H.   290
Hall, W.D.   3
Hammonds, Karl E.   157
Harburg, E.   13
Harrison, D.S.   322
Harrison, I.E.   322
Hartin, G.   154
Hatch, J.   148
Haughton, J.G.   158
Hawkins, R.   228
Haywood, L.J.   14, 15
Hebert, T.A.
Heisel, M.A.   70
Helfgott, M.A.   368
Helzer, J.E.   76
Henry, J.L.   190
Herman, K.D.   110
Heymsfield, S.   24
Hick, E.J.   355
Himes, J.H.   229
Hochbert, M.C.   230
Holliday, B.G.   159
Holmes, D.   231
Holtzman, N.A.   352

Horton, R.   355
Hosten, A.O.   16
Howze, D.C.   160
Huffine, C.L.   66
Hunter, K.I.   238

J

Jackson, J.J.   161
Jackson, J.S.   247
Jackson, R.K.   324
James, S.A.   17, 18, 249
Jeffrey, T.B.   128
Johnson, D.G.   239
Johnson, E.F.   162
Jones, B.E.   77, 78, 79, 80, 81
Jones, E.   82
Jones, J.H.   163
Jones, M.H.   68
Jones, R.L.   356
Jones, W., Jr.   83, 331, 332

K

Kail, B.B.   232
Kane, R.   164, 208
Kardiner, A.   84
Karp, R.J.   19
Kasl, S.V.   85
Kasteler, J.M.   164
Keil, J.E.   20
Keisling, R.   86
Keith, T.A.   21
Kerr, G.R.   22, 233
Khaton, O.M.   87
Kilgore, L.T.   219
Kiple, K.F.   325
Klein, H.E.   42
Kleiner, R.J.   106
Koegel, P.   88
Kong, B.W.   23
Kovi, J.   291
Kuller, L.   10

L

Lairson, D.   234
Lang, F.   357
Langford, H.G.   25

Lash, M.E.   1657
Lawson, W.B.   89
Leaverton, P.E.   26
Lee, A.S.   39
Lee, E.S.   126, 178, 235
LeFlore, I.C.   236
Levin, J.S.   166
Levy, D.R.   167
Lewis, D.O.   90
Lewis, E.A.   27
Lightfoot, O.B.   91, 168
Linde, S.M.   358
Linet, M.S.   230
Link, C.R.   237
Linn, B.S.   238
Linn, M.W.   238
Lloyd, S.M.   239
Locke, B.Z.   55
Long, S.H.   237
Lorimor, R.   234
Lothstein, L.M.   92
Lucas, F.   93
Luchins, D.J.   94
Lukoff, I.F.   232
Lyles, M.R.   95
Lynds, B.G.   28
Lythcott, G.I.   326

M

Markides, K.S.   169
Martin, B.J.W.   170
Matsuoka, L.Y.   292
Matthews, M.S.   359
Matthewson, M.A.   155
May, J.T.   240
Mayo, J.A.   96
Maypole, D.E.   171
McFalls, J.A.   241
McFarlane, J.   360
McGhee, N.   267
McShane, D.   242
Meagher, R.   71
Mears, G.J.   361
Medina, A.S.   243
Mehta, H.   47, 48
Mercer, K.   97
Merritt, L.   98
Messeri, P.   203

AUTHOR INDEX

Meyer, L.D. 244
Michielutte, R. 293
Miles, M.E. 327
Miller, C.A. 249
Miller, G.D. 355
Miller, J.M. 294
Miller, W.J. 295
Milner, M. 173
Mirowsky, J. 99
Molica, R.F. 100
Morgan, B.M. 28
Morgan, B.S. 245
Mukherjee, S. 101
Mumtax, F.B. 6
Munford, P.R. 102

N

Nace, E.P. 174
Nader, P.R. 139
National Center for Education
 In Maternal and Child Health 362
National League for Nursing 328
Neaton, J.D. 30
Neighbors, H.W. 103, 246, 247
Newmark, C.S. 104
Nurco, D.N. 248

O

Oberman, A. 31
Oliver, J. 6
Opler, M.K. 105
Orgue, M.S. 323
Orr, S.T. 249
Ory, H.W. 329
Osei, A. 156

P

Parker, S. 106
Parson, E.B. 81
Payne, L. 330
Payton, C.R. 107
Peck, D.L. 108
Pennici, E.A. 251
Peoples, M.D. 253
Peters, B.H. 351
Pierce, R.O. 252
Pierre, T. 32
Portnoi, V.A. 1755

Postell, W.D. 250
Pottern, L.M. 296
Pressior, R. 297
Pumariega, A.J. 109

R

Radford, E.P. 270
Rahbar, F. 176, 254
Raskin, A. 110
Redlich, F. 100
Reid, J.D. 177, 178
Reilly, P. 370
Reing, A.B. 363
Relman, A.S. 255
Remington, R.D. 33
Rene' A. 144, 179
Rice, H. 330
Rice, M.F. 180, 181, 331, 332
Ridley, C.R. 111
Ries, L.G. 298
Riggs, R.S. 182
Roback, H. 92
Roberts, R.E. 126, 127, 149
Robertson, H.R. 183
Robinson, J.C. 256
Rochat, R.W. 299
Rogers, E.L. 300
Rosen, T. 301
Rosenfield, S. 112
Ross, C.E. 99
Rostand, S.G. 257
Rothman, I. 216
Rowkema, R. 113
Rowland, M.L. 34
Royster, L.H. 212
Rozehort, R. 1
Ruffin, J.E. 333
Ruiz, D.S. 184
Ryder, N.B. 278

S

Sager, C.J. 114
Salber, E. 226, 258
Samuel-Reid, J.H. 364
Sargent, M.B. 259
Savitt, T. 260, 365
Schafft, G. 187, 188
Schatzkin, A. 334

Schmidt, R.M. 366
Schneller, E.S. 261
Schquer, P.K. 292
Schutte, J.E. 264
Schwartz, A.L. 367
Schwartz, B. 262
Scott, R.B. 368, 369
Seham, M. 185, 335
Sellers, R.V. 263
Settle, R.F. 237
Seyler, S.K. 28
Shader, R.I. 189
Shafer, S.Q. 265, 266
Shaffer, J.W. 248
Shah, N.D. 267
Shanok, S.S. 90
Shaw, C.T. 186
Silber, T.J. 115
Sills, E.M. 230
Simms, P. 70
Sinkford, J.C. 190
Sinnette, C.H. 308
Slater, C. 234
Smith, A., Jr. 116
Smith, E.J. 118
Smith, O.S. 118
Smith, R.J. 302
Smoyak, S.A. 268
Snow, L.F. 269
Southern Christian Leadership Conference 336
Spaulding, J.G. 140
Spirey, G.H. 270
Spollen, J.J. 210
Stamek, J. 4
Steele, M.F. 271
Steer, R.A. 119
Steinberg, A. 134
Steinberg, M.D. 120
Steinhorn, S.C. 303
Sterling, R.P. 35
Stokes, L. 337
Strong, J.P. 36
Sue, S. 121

T

Tebben, M.P. 37, 38
Terisi, J.A. 231
Termini, T.E. 272
Thomas, C.W. 122
Thompson, T. 338
Thornton, C.I. 123

Tolnay, S.E. 273
Tomelleri, C.J. 124
Tracy, M. 189
Tuckson, R. 274
Turner, T. 339

U

Uy, C.G. 369

V

Vail, A. 125
Vernon, S.W. 126, 127, 275

W

Walters, G.D. 128
Walters, I. 370
Wan, T.T. 276
Warnecke, R.B. 277
Watkins, B.A. 129
Watts, T.D. 191
Waxenburg, B.R. 114
Weaver, J.L. 192, 340, 341
Weiner, T.S. 261
Westoff, C.F. 278
Wethers, D.L. 344
White, E.H. 279, 342
White, J.E. 304
White, M.G. 130
Whitten, C.F. 371
Willenbring, M.L. 242
Williams, S.J. 131
Wilson, J.L. 193
Wilson, P.A. 194
Wilson, P.W. 39
Windham, F.
Wing, S. 280
Winn, M. 343
Wolf, A.M. 132
Wolf, J.H. 195
Wolinsky, F.D. 281
Wood, W.D. 133
Woolhandler, S. 282
Wright, R. 191

Y

Yabura, L. 196
Yamamoto, J. 134
Yankauer, A. 197
Yesavage, J.A. 89

AUTHOR INDEX

Yokie, A.J. 188
Young, J.L. 305, 306

Z

Zinkowski, J. 136
Ziff, M. 272